ECG
INTERPRETATION
made ridiculously simple

Michael A. Chizner, MD, FACP, FACC, FAHA

Founder and Former Chief Medical Director, The Heart Center of Excellence
Founding Director, Cardiology Fellowship Program
Broward Health
Fort Lauderdale, Florida

Clinical Professor of Medicine
University of Miami Miller School of Medicine
Miami, Florida

Clinical Professor of Medicine
University of Florida College of Medicine
Gainesville, Florida

Clinical Professor of Medicine
Dr. Kiran C. Patel College of Osteopathic Medicine at Nova Southeastern University
Fort Lauderdale, Florida

Clinical Professor of Integrated Medical Science
Charles E. Schmidt College of Medicine at Florida Atlantic University
Boca Raton, Florida

Clinical Professor of Medicine
Herbert Wertheim College of Medicine at Florida International University
Miami, Florida

Clinical Professor of Medicine
Barry University
Miami, Florida

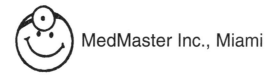

MedMaster Inc., Miami

ISBN #978-1-935660-42-2

Made in the United States of America

Published by MedMaster, Inc.
P.O. Box 640028
Miami, FL 33164

Cover and artwork by Richard March

Contents

Part I The Electrocardiogram (ECG)

Cardiac electrical activity and the ECG • The cardiac conduction system • ECG electrodes and leads

The standard 12-lead ECG • Rate and rhythm • The P wave • The QRS complex • The T wave • The U wave • The PR interval • The ST segment • The QT interval • QRS axis

Part II Major ECG Abnormalities: Diagnostic Clues and Clinical Correlations

Dedication

To my family …
without whose love, support,
and encouragement,
this book would not have been possible.

About the Author

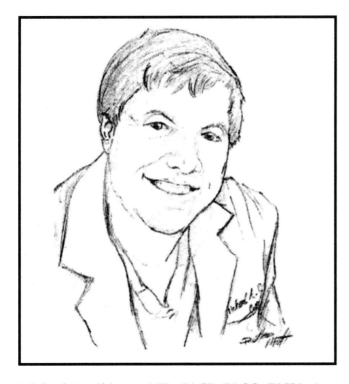

Michael A. Chizner, MD, FACP, FACC, FAHA, is a nationally renowned cardiologist, and the Founder and Former Chief Medical Director of The Heart Center of Excellence at Broward Health, one of the nation's largest health care systems based in Fort Lauderdale, Florida. He is a Clinical Professor of Medicine at the University of Florida College of Medicine, the University of Miami Miller School of Medicine, the Dr. Kiran C. Patel College of Osteopathic Medicine at Nova Southeastern University, the Charles E. Schmidt College of Medicine at Florida Atlantic University, the Herbert Wertheim College of Medicine at Florida International University, and Barry University.

Dr. Chizner graduated with highest honors from the Weill Cornell Medical College of Cornell University, where he was selected a member of the Alpha Omega Alpha National Medical Honor Society. He received his residency training in Internal Medicine at the New York Presbyterian Hospital-Weill Cornell Medical Center, and his cardiology fellowship training with legendary cardiologist W. Proctor Harvey, M.D., at Georgetown University, where he was the recipient of the Distinguished Alumnus Award. Dr. Chizner is a board-certified Diplomate of the American Board of Internal Medicine and the sub-specialty Board of Cardiovascular Disease. He is also a Fellow of the American College of Cardiology, the Council on Clinical Cardiology of the American Heart Association, and the American College of Physicians.

Dr. Chizner is a highly accomplished cardiac clinician-diagnostician, widely known for his clinical skills—especially in the art of auscultation—and his humanistic approach to patient care. Among the many awards and accolades he has received, Dr. Chizner has earned the distinction of being recognized as one of the top 1% of physicians in the nation in such prestigious publications as *America's Top Doctors, America's Top Cardiologists,*

America's Best Physicians, Who's Who in Medicine and Healthcare, Who's Who in America, U.S. News & World Report Top Doctors, and *The Leading Physicians of the World.* As physician, author, editor, and teacher, Dr. Chizner has contributed greatly to the practice of cardiology and the advancement of medical education. He has written and edited numerous articles, monographs, and books in cardiology, including the best-selling *Clinical Cardiology Made Ridiculously Simple,* that have become standards in cardiovascular education, and are now being used in medical schools throughout the United States and abroad.

Dr. Chizner has served on the editorial advisory boards of national cardiology journals. He has also been director, lecturer, and keynote speaker at continuing medical education conferences. Dr. Chizner has long been involved in the instruction of medical students, residents, fellows, physicians, nurses, and other healthcare professionals, and was the founding Director of the Cardiology Fellowship Program at Broward Health. In recognition of his outstanding achievements, Dr. Chizner received a gubernatorial appointment to the Florida Board of Medicine, where he served as Chairman of the Credentials Committee, and was elected unanimously by his fellow board members as Vice Chairman and Chairman of the Board. In honor of his hard work and lifelong dedication to his profession and his patients, Dr. Chizner was selected as the recipient of the prestigious *Who's Who* Albert Nelson Marquis Lifetime Achievement Award.

Preface

The electrocardiogram (ECG), introduced into clinical practice more than a century ago, remains one of the most important and widely used cardiac diagnostic tests in all of medicine. When performed in the appropriate clinical context, the information obtained from this simple, inexpensive, readily available, noninvasive tool often enables the well-trained clinician, skilled in the art of ECG interpretation, to make a rapid, accurate, and cost-effective cardiac diagnosis with fewer, if any, additional, more sophisticated and expensive laboratory tests.

Regrettably, in this age of advanced technology, ECG interpretation skills are inadequately emphasized both in education and practice. As a consequence, many of today's practitioners lack proficiency and confidence in interpreting ECGs (disuse atrophy) and rely too heavily on the computer-generated report, which is often inaccurate, to interpret their patient's ECG for them.

Computerized ECG analysis is no substitute for a solid foundation in clinical electrocardiography. Despite the increasing reliance on computer technology, it is still true that the well-trained clinician can derive a great deal of information about a patient's cardiovascular status by performing a careful and thoughtful interpretation of the ECG.

Accordingly, *ECG Interpretation Made Ridiculously Simple* is designed to provide present-day clinicians and trainees with a lucid, straightforward summary of the fundamental principles of ECG analysis and interpretation. Written by the clinician for the clinician, this handy study guide distills basic ECG concepts into a concise, clear, minimum, while including the essential information to read and interpret ECGs accurately and confidently.

The book is organized into two parts. The chapters in Part I present a brief overview of basic electrocardiography and a systematic approach to ECG interpretation. The chapters in Part II focus on the major ECG abnormalities encountered in clinical practice along with their diagnostic clues and clinical correlations. Pearls and pitfalls of ECG interpretation will also be discussed, along with the clinical indications and practical applications of the specialized ECG-based tools and techniques used in medicine and cardiology today. A concise yet comprehensive table of the most common ECG findings encountered in a wide variety of cardiac and noncardiac conditions is provided in the easily accessible, user-friendly Appendix. More than 50 case-based practice ECGs are also included to solidify key concepts, sharpen interpretation skills, test the reader's knowledge, and enhance understanding of the material presented in the book.

In addition to the easily readable text, the numerous ECG tracings, figures, and illustrative cartoons interspersed throughout the book serve as a visual aid to make the learning and understanding of ECG interpretation easy, memorable, and enjoyable. When more in-depth information is required, the reader is encouraged to refer to the companion text,

Clinical Cardiology Made Ridiculously Simple, now in its fifth edition.

It is my sincere hope that the information provided in this book will be extremely useful for Board preparation and course study, and prove to be of great value to all students and practitioners who strive to learn and master the "time-honored" art of ECG interpretation and become an *"Ace of Hearts."*

I welcome your comments and suggestions for future editions.

Michael A. Chizner, MD

Acknowledgments

I would like to express my deepest appreciation to the individuals whose help was invaluable in the preparation of this book.

I am extremely grateful to

- Dr. Stephen Goldberg, President of MedMaster, Inc., for his warm, continuing friendship and for providing me with expert assistance and guidance on how to "keep it ridiculously simple."
- Mr. Richard March, illustrator and cartoonist extraordinaire, whose exceptional artistic skills helped to pictorially "bring to life" the material presented in the text.
- Ms. Phyllis Goldenberg, for her helpful suggestions and detailed proofreading of the text.
- Ms. Stephanie Crossley, my office manager, whose superb administrative skills, along with her meticulous attention to detail and her ability to multitask were essential to bringing this book to fruition.

- Mrs. Aniamma Geevarghese, APRN, Mrs. Kelly M. Roland, APRN, Mrs. Beth Brand, and Ms. Carly Yeckes for their unrelenting enthusiasm, dedication, and faithful support.
- The many medical students, residents, fellows, physicians, nurses, and other health care professionals with whom I have had the pleasure and privilege to work, for inspiring me and for making the teaching and learning of clinical cardiology so meaningful and enjoyable.

And especially to

- My devoted and loving family – my wife Susan, and our children Kevin, Ryan, Blair and Jon; my sister Joan; and in loving memory of my mother Sybil and my father Bernard – without whom this book would not have been possible.

A "simple" thank you will never be enough!

Michael A. Chizner, MD

Part I. The Electrocardiogram

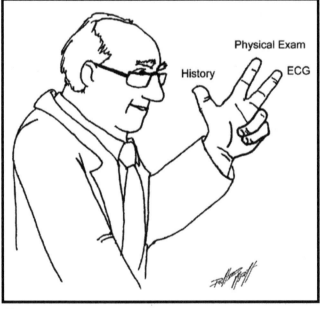

Fig. I-1.

The evaluation of a patient with cardiac disease proceeds through an orderly sequence of events that begins with a careful clinical history and physical examination. The electrocardiogram (ECG) is then performed, as needed, and the results integrated into an assessment of the probability of cardiovascular disease (**Figure I-1**).

Despite today's advanced technology, the simple 12-lead ECG remains a cornerstone of the clinical cardiologic evaluation. This readily available, point-of-care test can be obtained easily and rapidly, is noninvasive and inexpensive, poses no risk to the patient, and can be read and interpreted immediately by trained personnel. Above all, the ECG remains a highly useful tool in assessing myocardial ischemia and/or infarction, cardiac arrhythmias and conduction disturbances, cardiac chamber enlargement and hypertrophy, pericarditis, metabolic and electrolyte imbalances, drug-induced effects, electronic pacemaker function, and other noncardiac conditions. Indeed, it is considered the test of "first choice" in the evaluation and management of patients who present with chest pain, palpitations, dizziness, or syncope.

Keep in mind, however, that the 12-lead ECG is only a diagnostic tool and like any tool in medicine, its clinical utility is critically dependent on an accurate interpretation. Computer ECG analysis may be subject to error. Errors in ECG interpretation can lead to misdiagnosis and inappropriate treatment. Careful over-reading by a skilled ECG interpreter, therefore, is essential.

The following chapters will present a brief overview of basic electrocardiography along with a stepwise, systematic approach to ECG interpretation. Once the basics of ECG analysis are understood and practiced in a repetitive manner, confidence in your ability to correctly identify normal and abnormal ECG findings improves significantly.

1

Basic Electrocardiography

A basic knowledge of the electrical activity of the heart is an essential requisite to understanding and interpreting the electrocardiogram (ECG). Although ECG interpretation may seem difficult at first, a clear understanding of relatively simple electrophysiologic principles will enable you to read and interpret ECGs more easily and accurately.

Cardiac Electrical Activity and the ECG

The electrocardiogram (simply ECG or EKG, short for "electrokardiogram") is a graphic display of the heart's electrical activity recorded from electrodes (sensors) placed on the patient's chest wall and extremities. It records two basic electrical processes:

1. *Depolarization* (the spread of electrical current through the heart muscle), producing the P wave from the atria and the QRS complex from the ventricles
2. *Repolarization* (the return of the stimulated muscle to the resting state), producing the ST segment, T wave and U wave. (**Figure 1-1**)

Figure 1-1. Basic components of the ECG. By convention, the ECG tracing is divided into the P wave, PR interval, QRS complex, QT interval, ST segment, T wave, and U wave.

These processes occur as charged particles called *ions* (sodium, potassium, and calcium) flow back and forth across cell membranes to generate an electrical impulse known as the *action potential* that stimulates the heart muscle to contract. The process whereby an action potential triggers heart muscle cells to contract is called *excitation-contraction coupling*.

An understanding of the mechanisms by which action potentials are generated and propagated through cardiac cells facilitates learning about the basic components of the surface ECG.

Figure 1-2. Left. Relationship of the phases (0-4) of a cardiac action potential from a ventricular muscle cell (top) to the cardiac electrical activity on the surface ECG (bottom).

Top. In a resting (or polarized) muscle cell (phase 4), sodium (Na^+) and calcium (Ca^{++}) ions, located on the outside of the cell, are unable to cross the cell wall. Potassium (K^+) ions, located on the inside of the cell, leak slowly across the cell wall to the outside. The charge on the outside of the muscle cell is positive, and the charge on the inside is negative. The resulting voltage difference across the cell membrane is called the *resting transmembrane potential* (which is approximately -90 mV). When the muscle cell is stimulated (phase 0), Na^+ ions rush into the cell through voltage-dependent pathways called *fast channels*, and Ca^{++} ions enter the cell through pathways called *slow channels*. The charge on the inside of the cell changes from negative to positive, and depolarization begins. A wave of depolarization then spreads from cell to cell through the entire heart. The waveforms recorded on the ECG represent depolarization of the muscle cells.

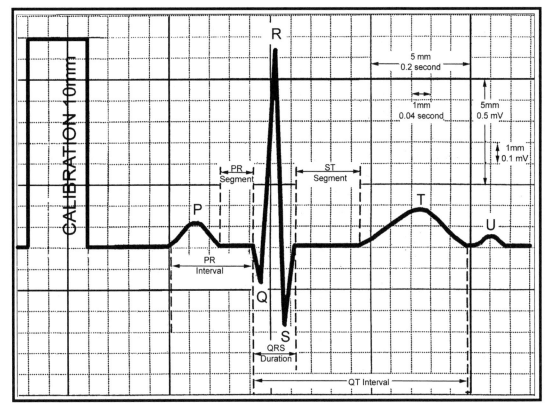

Fig. 1-1.

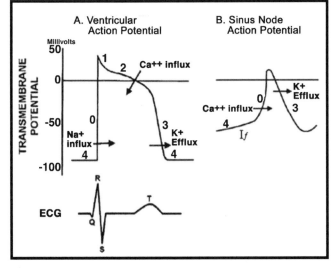

Fig. 1-2.

In the muscle cells of the atrium, phase 0 of the action potential (depolarization) correlates with the P wave on the ECG (not shown here).

Bottom. In the muscle cells of the ventricles, phase 0 of the action potential (depolarization) correlates with the QRS complex on the ECG. Phases 1, 2, and 3 of the action potential represent repolarization, or recovery of the cells. The inside of the cell changes from positive back to its original resting negative charge. During phase 1, the fast sodium channels suddenly close, while the slow calcium channels remain open. During phase 2, the continued flow of Ca^{++} into the cell is balanced by the flow of K^+ to the outside of the cell. Phase 2 correlates with the ST segment on the ECG. During phase 3, the calcium channels close while K^+ continues to leak to the outside. Phase 3 correlates with the T wave on the ECG. After depolarization, there is a period of time called the *refractory period* during which the muscle cell cannot depolarize again. There are two parts to the refractory period. The absolute refractory period is the time when the muscle cell cannot respond to any other stimuli. The relative refractory period is the time toward the end of repolarization when the muscle cell can potentially respond if the stimulus is strong enough. Such a recovery period is physiologically necessary because it allows the ventricles sufficient time to relax and refill before the next contraction. When the recovery (or repolarization) process has been completed, the cell is ready to be activated, or depolarized again. While depolarization spreads through the ventricular wall from endocardium (the inner layer) to epicardium (the outer layer), repolarization proceeds from epicardium to endocardium. As a result, the T wave (repolarization) is normally inscribed on the ECG in the same direction as the QRS complex (depolarization) because a negative electrical current moving away from a recording electrode is perceived as a positive electrical current moving toward it (i.e., a double negative equals a positive). The T wave is normally broader than the QRS complex, however, because the wave of repolarization is more diffuse and travels less rapidly than the wave of depolarization.

Right. Sinus node action potential. Not all cardiac cells rely on an electrical stimulus for initial depolarization. In sinus node (shown here) and AV nodal cells, spontaneous diastolic (phase 4) depolarization is mediated by a slow inward movement of sodium ions that enter the cell through unique voltage gated channels called *funny channels* (I*f*), which open in response to hyperpolarization (a state in which the interior of the cell is very negative). I*f* channels begin to open when the membrane potential becomes more negative than approximately -50 mV. The inward flow of positively charged sodium ions through the funny channels causes the membrane potential to become progressively less negative, ultimately depolarizing the cell to its threshold voltage. When the critical threshold voltage is reached, phase 0 of the action potential begins as calcium ions enter the cell through relatively slow calcium channels.

In contrast to the heart muscle cells, sinus node and AV nodal cells (so-called *pacemaker cells*) are able to generate an action potential independently from any other cells. This innate ability to spontaneously depolarize is known as *automaticity*. The sinoatrial (SA) node is the primary pacemaker site within the heart and establishes the normal electrical pattern known as *sinus rhythm*. The repolarization phase of pacemaker cells results from both the inactivation of the open calcium channels and the opening of voltage gated potassium channels that permit efflux of K$^+$ from the cells.

The Cardiac Conduction System

After depolarization and repolarization occur, the resulting electrical impulse travels through the heart along a pathway called the conduction system. The prime function of the cardiac conduction system is to transmit electrical impulses from the sinoatrial (SA) node (where they are normally generated) to the atria and ventricles, causing them to contract.

Figure 1-3. The cardiac conduction system. During each cardiac cycle, an electrical impulse is generated by the sinoatrial (SA) node, the heart's primary pacemaker, which is located in the right atrium near the entry of the superior vena cava. The SA node spontaneously depolarizes at a rate of 60-100 times/minute. The SA node is susceptible to influence from the parasympathetic nervous system via the vagus nerve (which slows heart rate) and the sympathetic nervous system (which increases heart rate). The

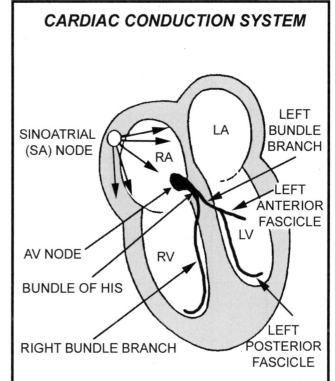

CARDIAC CONDUCTION SYSTEM

Fig. 1-3.

impulse travels to atrial myocardial muscle cells by way of three internodal tracts (anterior, middle, and posterior) in the right atrium, and an additional pathway called *Bachmann's bundle* in the left atrium, causing a wave of atrial muscle cell depolarization. The electrical impulse briefly slows at the AV node, delaying ventricular activity and allowing blood from the atrial contraction to fill the ventricles. From the AV node, the impulse passes extremely rapidly through the bundle of His to the right and left bundle branches and to the Purkinje fibers, which trigger ventricular muscle cell depolarization and then contraction of the ventricles. The electrical activity of the SA node, AV node, bundle of His, and Purkinje fibers does not show up on the ECG. Rather, it is the actual depolarization of myocardial fibers (the so-called *working* [contracting] *cells*) that shows up. In the absence of an SA node, the AV node will drive the heartbeat, albeit at a slower rate than normal (40-60 beats per minute). In the absence of the SA and AV node functions, a slower ventricular rhythm will prevail (20-40 beats per minute). Normally, these slower potential pacemaker sites (*ectopic foci*) in the AV node and ventricle are suppressed by the faster rate of the dominant SA node. This is known as *overdrive suppression*. These backup mechanisms (so-called *escape rhythms*) are a form of "safety net" to help ensure that the ventricles will continue beating in the presence of defects to SA and/or AV nodal discharges.

The ECG provides three pieces of information about the electrical activity generated by the heart during the cardiac cycle: *duration, amplitude,* and *direction* (electrical axis).

The *duration* is the time required to depolarize (or repolarize) various structures. At a standard paper speed of 25 mm/sec, each small box (1 mm) horizontally on the ECG paper represents 0.04 seconds, and each large box (5 mm) represents 0.20 seconds. (**Figure 1-1**) Abnormal duration may indicate impairment of electrical propagation.

The *amplitude* of the electrical activity is expressed in millivolts and is measured by the vertical markings on the ECG paper. When the ECG machine is set at "standard," each millimeter of amplitude equals 0.1 mV (10 mm = 1 mV). (**Figure 1-1**). Voltage is determined in part by the size of the cardiac chambers as well as the body habitus and various pathological conditions.

The *direction* of electrical activity refers to the overall vector direction of electrical depolarization of the ventricular myocardium. Many abnormalities affect the direction of electrical activity produced by depolarization as well as repolarization.

Figure 1-4. The overall direction of ventricular myocardial cell depolarization normally spreads downward (inferiorly) and to the (patient's) left (since the left ventricle is much larger and has more muscle mass than the right ventricle) and is referred to as the *axis of depolarization.* The axis may point outside the patient's lower left quadrant in different pathological states, either to the patient's right side (right axis deviation) or the patient's left upper quadrant (left axis deviation).

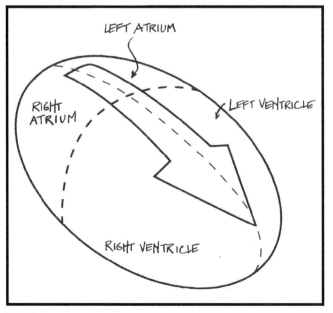

Fig. 1-4.

(From Goldberg, S. *Clinical Physiology Made Ridiculously Simple,* MedMaster, Inc., 2014)

ECG Electrodes and Leads

ECG electrodes are conductive pads (sensors) that are attached to the skin surface and detect electrical currents. Where and how ECG electrodes are placed on the body are critical determinants of the morphology of the ECG signal. A pair of ECG electrodes constitutes an ECG lead. Each ECG lead provides a unique view of the heart's electrical activity. The "standard" ECG consists of 12 different leads (electrode connections) used to provide a complete panoramic picture of the heart's electrical activity as seen from different angles. The 12-lead ECG is generated from 10 electrodes; 4 attached to the extremities, 1 of which is a ground (not shown in **Figure 1-5**), produce 6 limb leads and 6 attached to the chest wall produce 6 precordial leads.

Figure 1-5. Attachments and viewing angles of the limb and chest leads. (From Goldberg, S. *Clinical Physiology Made Ridiculously Simple,* MedMaster, Inc., 2014)

- Six leads that are derived from the electrodes placed on the arms and left leg are called *extremity* or *limb leads*: 3 bipolar leads (I, II, and III), and 3 unipolar augmented leads (augmented vector right [aVR], augmented vector left [aVL], and augmented vector foot [aVF]). These 6 leads register the direction, amplitude, and duration of the heart's electrical activity, as seen from 6 different positions in the frontal plane (picture a flat plane lying on the patient's chest).

- The 6 remaining leads are called *precordial* or *chest leads* (V1 to V6). These leads provide information about the heart's electrical activity in the horizontal plane (picture a flat plane crossing through the patient's chest).

Each ECG lead provides a different view of the heart's electrical activity between two points or poles (a positive pole and a negative pole). The direction in which the electric current flows determines how the waveforms appear on the ECG tracing.

- The 3 bipolar limb leads I, II, and III, introduced by Einthoven, record the difference in electrical potential between the right arm (−) and left arm (+) for lead I; right arm (−) and left leg (+) for lead II; and left arm (−) and left leg (+) for lead III (**Figure 1-5**). An electrode is also attached to the patient's right leg, but this serves only as an electrical ground that helps prevent electrical interference from appearing on the ECG, and is not an active recording site.

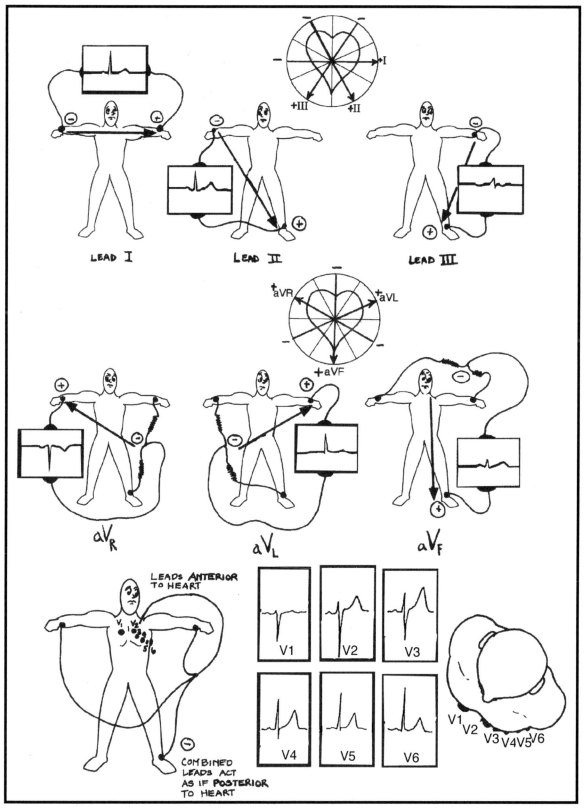

Fig. 1-5.

- The 3 unipolar limb leads, aVR, aVL and aVF, designed by Goldberger, are termed unipolar since there is a single positive limb electrode that is referenced against a combination of the other two limb electrodes, which serve as the negative pole of that pair. Unipolar limb leads are called *augmented leads* because the ECG machine must amplify the voltage in order to get adequate recordings. Lead aVR is created by making the electrode on the right arm positive. The electrodes on the left arm and left leg serve as a common ground and are both negative. Lead aVL is created by making the electrode on the left arm positive. The electrodes on the right arm and left leg serve as a common ground and are both negative. Lead aVF is created by making the electrode on the left leg positive. The electrodes on the right arm and left arm serve as a common ground and are both negative (**Figure 1-5**). Keep in mind that the positive poles of limb leads I, II, III, aVL, and aVF are positioned on the body surface to the left and inferiorly, whereas the positive pole of lead aVR is positioned on the right.

If a wave of depolarization is moving toward a positive electrode, this is reflected in a positive (upward) movement of the wave on the ECG recording. If the wave of depolarization is moving away from a positive electrode, this results in a negative (downward) deflection of the wave on the ECG recording. Normally, there is a positive deflection in leads I, II, III, aVL and aVF because depolarization is moving inferiorly and to the (patient's) left, toward the positive electrodes. Conversely, there is a negative deflection in lead aVR because depolarization is moving away from the positive electrode. Leads I and aVL are called the *lateral leads* since they best measure electrical activity on the left side of the heart. Leads II, III, and aVF are called the *inferior leads* since they best measure electrical activity on the underside of the heart. Lead aVR best measures electrical activity on the right side of the heart (**Figure 1-6**).

Figure 1-6. The viewpoint each limb lead has of the heart. The limb leads look at the heart from a different angle in the frontal plane.

For the chest leads (V1-V6), the negative pole is generated by combining all 3 limb electrodes together (a virtual reference point known as *Wilson's central terminal*). Each of the 6 chest leads uses the relevant chest electrode as the positive pole.

Figure 1-7. The viewpoint each chest lead has of the heart. The chest leads look at the heart from a different angle in the horizontal plane.

The 6 unipolar precordial leads are placed as follows: V1, the fourth intercostal space to the right of the sternum; V2, the fourth intercostal space to the left of the sternum; V3, midway between leads V2 and

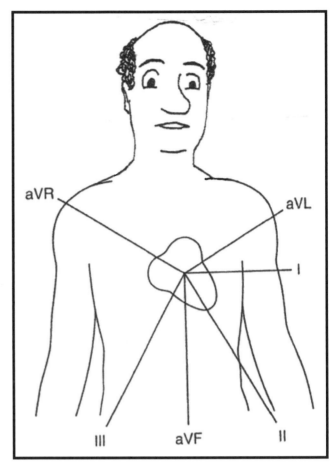

Fig. 1-6.

V4. Lead V4 is placed in the fifth intercostal space at the midclavicular line, V5 is placed between V4 and V6, and V6 is placed at the midaxillary line at the level of lead V4. These 6 leads are all positive, with the negative electrode being the combined limb leads (accomplished by internal connections in the ECG machine). Normally, the QRS complex begins with a predominantly negative (downward) deflection in V1 and V2 because depolarization is traveling away from the positive electrodes. The QRS complex ends with a predominantly positive (upward) deflection in V5 and V6 because depolarization is traveling toward the positive electrodes.

Leads V1 and V2 provide a view of the interventricular septum; leads V3 and V4 of the anterior wall of the left ventricle; and leads V5 and V6 (along with leads I and aVL) of the lateral aspect of the left ventricle. Lead V1 lies anteriorly and medially over the right ventricle, and along with aVR is referred to as the right ventricular leads.

Confused? The preceding discussion can be difficult to go through. You may want to simply memorize the following generalities before proceeding;

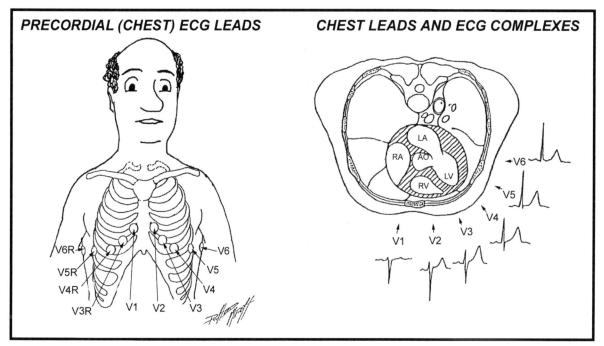

Fig. 1-7.

The ECG records the electrical activity of the heart from electrodes placed on the surface of the body. The ECG leads (electrode connections) are designed to look at the heart from different angles:

- Leads I and aVL look at the left side of the heart. ("L" = "left")
- Leads II, III, and aVF look at the inferior (diaphragmatic) side of the heart ("F" = "foot")
- Lead aVR looks at the right side of the heart. ("R" = "right")
- The 6 precordial leads (V1-V6) look at the anterior and lateral sides of the heart from right to left.

Knowing the viewpoint of each lead allows you to determine which areas of the heart are affected by, for example, a myocardial infarction. An inferior wall MI will produce changes in the leads looking at that area, namely leads II, III, and aVF. An anterior MI produces changes mainly in leads V1-V4. and a lateral wall MI produces changes in leads I, aVL, V5 and V6.

In certain circumstances, additional chest leads not part of the "standard" 12-lead ECG may be used to view specific areas of the heart. Right-sided chest leads (particularly V4R), placed in a "mirror image" pattern to the normal left-sided chest leads, can provide a clue to RV infarction (**Figure 1-7**). Posterior chest leads (V7, V8, and V9), placed in the posterior axillary, mid scapular, and left paraspinal lines respectively, can help confirm the diagnosis of a posterior MI.

2

A Systematic Approach to ECG Interpretation

There are several general approaches to interpreting ECGs. One is the *pattern recognition method*, where you commit all possible patterns to memory, and then study each ECG for the presence of these patterns. If you have perfect memory, and are always presented with classic ("textbook") ECGs, this approach may be reasonable. However, many patients "don't read the textbook." Another (perhaps more practical and logical) method is to take a systematic, *step-by-step approach*, so that nothing is overlooked, as follows:

- First check the *basics* (e.g., correct patient name and date, standard voltage calibration).
- Determine the *heart rate* and *rhythm*.
- Evaluate the mean directional electrical *QRS axis*.
- Examine each *interval* (PR, QRS, QT) and *wave* or *complex* (P, QRS, ST, and T).

Put this information together and assess it for signs of cardiac arrhythmias and conduction disturbances, chamber enlargement and hypertrophy, myocardial ischemia and/or infarction, as well as drug effects and metabolic and electrolyte abnormalities, interpreting them in light of the clinical context (i.e., patient's age, presenting complaint, and additional relevant clinical history).

Skilled interpretation of the ECG requires a careful and thoughtful approach. Keep in mind the mnemonic "**BRAICE**" yourself: **B**asics, **R**ate and rhythm, **A**xis, **I**ntervals, **C**onformations (morphology) of the waves and complexes, **E**verything else when reading an ECG.

With repeated practice, you may begin to master the essentials of ECG interpretation.

The Standard 12-Lead ECG

Let us now correlate the electrical activity in the heart with the inscriptions ("squiggly lines") they make on the standard 12-lead ECG. By convention, the letters P, Q, R, S, T, and U are used to designate the six major waves or deflections of the ECG. The P, T, and U waves are represented by upper case letters. Lower case letters are often used to describe the Q, R, and S waves, depending on their relative or absolute size. The P-QRS-T complex of the normal ECG represents electrical activity over one cardiac cycle.

- The *P wave* indicates atrial depolarization. (The firing of the SA node does not give a strong enough signal to be detected on the ECG.)
- The *QRS complex* indicates ventricular depolarization. The QRS complex is normally larger than the P wave because depolarization of the greater muscle mass of the ventricles generates more voltage than does depolarization of the thinner walls of the atria.
- The *T wave* represents ventricular repolarization. (The wave of atrial repolarization is not detected normally since it is usually hidden within the large QRS complex of ventricular depolarization.)

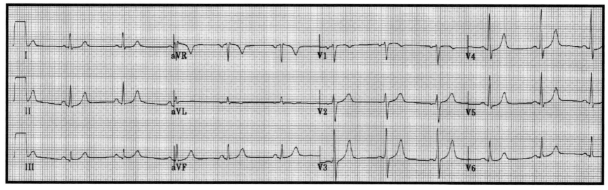

Fig. 2-1.

- A *U wave* (not always seen) follows the T wave and indicates poorly understood ventricular afterpotentials.
- The *PR interval* is the time between the beginning of the P wave and the beginning of the QRS. It is the time between the onset of atrial depolarization and the onset of ventricular depolarization. It is commonly used as an estimation of AV nodal conduction time, since most of this interval is spent in the delay traversing the AV node.
- The *ST segment* is the segment between the end of the QRS interval and the beginning of the T wave. It is the pause between the end of ventricular depolarization and the beginning of ventricular repolarization.
- The *QT interval* (the time between the beginning of the QRS and the end of the T wave) represents the total duration of both ventricular depolarization and repolarization. (**Note:** A *segment* is a stretch of baseline. An *interval* includes at least one wave.)

Familiarize yourself with the order in which the leads are arranged on the ECG tracing. On the left side of the tracing (first and second columns) are the limb leads I, II, III and aVR, aVL, aVF, respectively. On the right side of the tracing (third and fourth columns) are the precordial (chest) leads V1, V2, V3 and V4, V5, V6, respectively. Getting accustomed to the layout of the tracing will help you interpret the ECG more quickly and accurately. Check the ECG tracing to see if it is technically correct (i.e., voltage calibration, proper lead placement). Make sure the baseline is free from electrical interference and drift. On some ECGs, a computer generated "reading" will also be displayed at the top of the tracing. These interpretations are not infallible. Always read and interpret the ECG yourself, then compare your findings. Focus on learning what each of the waves, segments, and intervals of the ECG represent and their normal appearance.

Figure 2-1. The normal 12-Lead ECG consists of the following waves, segments and intervals:

- The *P wave*, a record of atrial depolarization, is upright in lead I, II, aVF; typically inverted in aVR; and may be inverted or biphasic in III, aVR, V1 and V2.
- The *PR interval*, the interval from the beginning of the P wave to the beginning of the QRS complex, is normally 0.12–0.20 seconds. It reflects the time required for conduction of the impulse through the atria, AV node, bundle of His, and bundle branches up to the time of ventricular depolarization.
- The *QRS interval*, the interval from the beginning of the Q wave to the end of the S wave, is usually 0.06–0.10 seconds. It reflects ventricular depolarization. The precordial transition zone (midpoint between negative and positive deflections) usually occurs between V3 and V4.
- *Q waves* are typical in leads aVR, V1 and V2. However, small q waves (<0.04 seconds in duration and height <25% of R wave) are common in most leads due to normal left to right septal depolarization, and should not be confused with old MI.
- The *ST segment*, the segment between the end of the QRS interval and the beginning of the T wave, is usually isoelectric. It may vary from 0.5 mm below to 1 mm above baseline in the limb leads. Up to 3 mm concave upward (valley-like) elevation in precordial leads may be seen (*early repolarization*).
- The *T wave* reflects ventricular repolarization. It is upright in leads I, II, V3–V6; typically inverted in aVR and V1; may be variable (upright, flat, inverted, or biphasic) in III, aVL, aVF, V1 and V2. T wave inversion in V1–V3 may be seen in healthy young adults (*persistent juvenile pattern*).
- The *QT interval*, the interval between the beginning of the QRS and the end of the T wave, represents

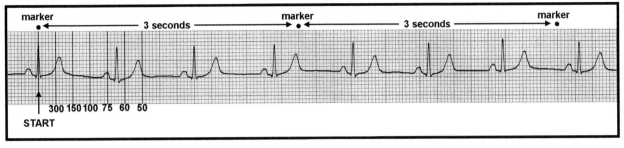

Fig. 2-2.

the duration of ventricular electrical activity, and corrected for heart rate (see below) is usually 0.44 seconds (in men) and 0.46 seconds (in women). It varies inversely with heart rate. (Roughly, if the heart rate is between 60 and 100, the QT interval should be less than 1/2 of the R-R interval, the interval between 2 consecutive R waves).

- The *U wave* is a small deflection following the T wave. It is usually, but not always, observed in the precordial leads, and may be due to repolarization of the bundle branches and Purkinje fibers.

Note: The rectangular upward deflection at the beginning of the ECG tracing is the voltage calibration signal (10 boxes = 1 mV). Each small box on the ECG grid is 0.04 seconds.

A patient's ECG can tell you much about the heart's depolarization-repolarization cycle.

Rate and Rhythm

Determining the heart rate and rhythm are the first two steps you should complete in every ECG interpretation. Although the ECG computer's calculation of the heart rate is generally accurate, artifact (e.g., muscle tremor), large T waves, and pacemaker spikes can confuse the computer and cause it to report an inaccurate rate.

A normal cardiac rhythm (normal sinus rhythm, NSR) is present if the heart rate is between 60 and 100 beats per minute and if every P wave is followed by a QRS; every QRS is preceded by a P wave; the P wave is upright in leads I, II and III (indicating that the P wave is originating from the sinus node); and the PR interval is > 0.12 seconds. The heart rate can be estimated in several ways:

- The simplest method is to find an R wave that lands on a heavy black line. Then count the number of large boxes to the next R wave. Count "300-150-100" and then "75-60-50" as each large box goes by until you get to the next R wave, thus providing an estimate of the heart rate (**Figure 2-2**). Alternatively, you may divide 300 by the number

of large boxes (or divide 1500 by the number of small boxes) between R waves.
- If the heart rate is less than 60, the above method may not be accurate. In that case, simply count the number of R waves in a 6-second strip and multiply by 10 (or in a 10-second ECG tracing and multiply by 6). This method is also useful if there is an irregular rhythm, where the distances between R waves may vary and you need a number of R waves to average out the measurement.

Figure 2-2. Estimating heart rate on the ECG. Count the number of QRS complexes between 3 markers (6 seconds) and multiply by 10. A similar rate is obtained using the "(300-150-100)(75-60-50)" method. In this case, the ventricular rate, as measured by the QRS complexes, is about 60–70.

Figure 2-3. A. Normal sinus rhythm (NSR).
B. A sinus rhythm that is slow (<60 beats/min) is a *sinus bradycardia* (some references use <50 beats/min).
C. A sinus rhythm that is fast (>100 beats/min), is a *sinus tachycardia.*
D. If the SA node fails, a backup pacemaker may arise in the AV node or proximal bundle of His, conducting at about 40–60 beats/min. This is termed a *junctional escape rhythm* or *idiojunctional rhythm.* There may not be a visible P wave, or there may be an inverted P wave either before or after the QRS complex, reflecting retrograde conduction of the P wave.
E. Failing that, the rhythm may be paced by the ventricles at about 20–40/min, termed a *ventricular escape rhythm* or *idioventricular rhythm.* Note the wide QRS arising from a pacemaker focus in the myocardium.

The term *supraventricular tachycardia* refers to tachycardias that are "above the ventricles," i.e., that are not ventricular in origin. They include atrial tachycardias as well as those originating within the AV node.

In normal sinus rhythm, the distance between the QRS complexes varies somewhat with respiration, the rate increasing slightly with the effort of inspiration (which

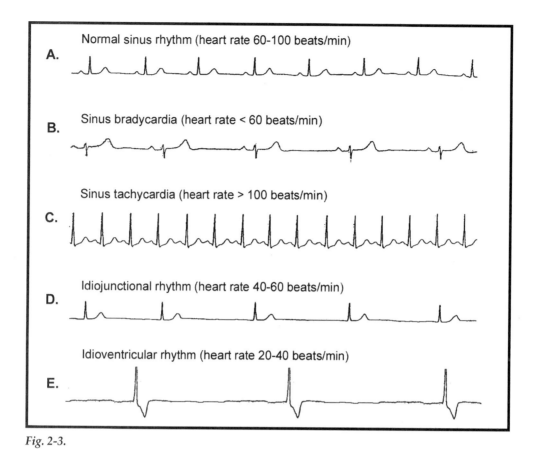

Fig. 2-3.

stretches the lung tissue and causes a reflex inhibition of vagal tone) and decreasing with the passive process of expiration (*sinus arrhythmia*). Sinus arrhythmia is a normal finding in healthy young adults and should not be confused with the more serious disturbances of cardiac conduction.

Rhythms other than NSR are termed *arrhythmias* (also known as *dysrhythmias*). Some arrhythmias are regular rhythms, but just slow (<60 beats/min) or fast (>100 beats/min), where the QRS complexes appear at regular intervals. Some rhythms are regularly irregular, i.e., have a recurrent pattern (e.g., Wenckebach phenomenon, where the QRS complexes get progressively farther apart, skip a beat, and then start all over closer together), while others are irregularly irregular, i.e., completely disorganized (e.g., atrial fibrillation, where the distances between QRS complexes have no regularity). It is important to ascertain whether an arrhythmia originates from the atria, ventricles, or conduction system that connects the atria and ventricles. This can make an important difference in understanding the underlying pathology and planning a therapeutic approach.

Diagnosing the origin of an ECG rate and rhythm often depends on a careful analysis of the individual ECG components, which will be discussed in **Chapter 5** on arrhythmias.

The P Wave

The P wave represents depolarization of atrial muscle cells. It results from sequential activation of the right atrium (where the SA node is located) and the left atrium. P wave morphology is best assessed in leads II and VI. A small, upright, rounded P wave (as seen in lead II) represents normal atrial depolarization. P wave abnormalities may deviate from the normal with respect to their location, amplitude (voltage), duration, positive or negative deflection, or contour (configuration).

Figure 2-4. In *right atrial enlargement* (also called *right atrial abnormality*), the P wave in lead II is tall (>2.5 mm) and pointed. The amplitude of the right atrial component of the P wave in lead V1 is increased, seen as an enlargement of the first part of the curve, since right atrial depolarization slightly precedes left atrial depolarization. Such a P wave is called *P pulmonale* since it is typically associated with chronic pulmonary disease, pulmonary embolism, and cor pulmonale.

In *left atrial enlargement* (also called *left atrial abnormality*), the P wave in lead II is broad and notched (*double hump*), and the terminal downward deflection of the biphasic P wave in lead V1 is increased in amplitude and duration (>1 mm wide

	Lead II	Lead V$_1$
NORMAL		
RA enlargement ("P Pulmonale")	 Tall P Wave (>2.5mm)	 Tall P Wave
LA enlargement ("P Mitrale")	 Broad & Notched P Wave	Wide & Deep Biphasic P Wave

Fig. 2-4.

and >1 mm deep) reflecting the later depolarization of the left atrium. Such a P wave is called *P mitrale* because it may result from volume and/or pressure overload of the left atrium as seen with mitral valve disease. Other common causes include LV hypertrophy (due to hypertension, AS, HOCM) and abnormal intra-atrial conduction. Because conditions other than *enlargement* cause P wave changes, the term *abnormality* is commonly used to designate alterations in P wave morphology.

If the P wave is negative in leads I or II, you should keep in mind three possibilities: inadvertent limb lead reversal, dextrocardia, and junctional rhythm (where the AV node pathologically is the pacemaker, and impulses spread backwards from the AV node to depolarize the atria).

The QRS Complex

The QRS complex results from the nearly simultaneous depolarization of both the right and left ventricles. The Q wave (due to normal left to right septal activation) is the first downward deflection of the QRS complex. Whether this is a downward deflection or an upward deflection depends on which side of the septum (left versus right respectively) a lead is "looking from" (i.e., small q wave in leads V5 and V6, small r wave in leads V1 and V2). It is followed by an upward R wave, and then a downward S wave. This total QRS complex represents the electrical activity of ventricular depolarization. The normal QRS complex is predominantly positive (above the baseline) in leads that "look" at the heart from the left side (I, aVL,

V5–V6) and in leads that "look" at the inferior surface of the heart (II, III, aVF). It is negative (below the baseline) in leads that "look" at the heart from the right side (aVR, V1–V2). The QRS complex is biphasic (part above and part below the baseline) in leads V3–V4. The process whereby the R wave becomes progressively taller from lead V1 through lead V6 is known as *R wave progression*. If there is only a single downward deflection with no R wave, then you cannot know whether to call the deflection a Q wave or an S wave, so it is termed a *QS wave*.

The QRS *width* (interval) normally is 0.10 seconds or less and should be examined for possible conduction abnormalities. The ECG demonstrates widening of the QRS and other changes representing interference with conduction when there is a delay or block of conduction in either the right or left bundles. It is better to evaluate QRS width in the limb leads than in the chest leads, since the amplitude of the QRS is generally higher in the chest leads, and a lag in ability of the ECG pen to write quickly may artifactually widen the QRS in the chest leads.

In *right bundle branch block* (RBBB), there is blockage of transmission of electrical information through the right bundle branch to the right ventricle myocardium. As a result, information has to take a divergent route from the left side of the heart to the right side, resulting in a delay of appearance of the right ventricle QRS. The QRS complexes of the right and left ventricles normally overlap to form a single QRS, but in RBBB the right ventricle QRS appears slightly after the start of the left ventricle QRS, resulting in an abnormally widened QRS

(>0.12 sec) with two R wave peaks, often called *R* and *R prime* (seen best in lead V1). In RBBB the QRS looks like an "M" or *rabbit ear pattern* in lead V1. In *left bundle branch block* (LBBB) there is a similar widening of the QRS, but it is the left ventricular QRS, which occupies the later part of the abnormally widened QRS. It too is often, but not always, notched at the top. In LBBB, the QRS looks like an "M" in lead V6. **Figure 2-5** compares typical RBBB with LBBB. Note that RBBB shows the "M" on the right side of the precordial leads (V1) and LBBB shows the "M" on the left side (V6). If you simply remember *right on the right* and *left on the left*, you can easily distinguish between the two.

Bundle branch block patterns with a QRS duration of 0.12 second or more are designated as complete and those with a QRS duration less than 0.12 seconds as incomplete.

Figure 2-5. Top. Right bundle branch block (RBBB). Note that the QRS is prolonged (>0.12 seconds), and the terminal positive wave is inscribed in lead V1 (rSR′ – *rabbit ear pattern*), since V1 lies on the right side and "sees" the RBBB delay moving toward it. Conversely, in lead V6, the delay is moving away from the electrode, producing a terminal wide negative S wave.

Bottom. Left bundle branch block (LBBB). Note the QRS is prolonged with a slurred upright R wave in lead V6 (the delay is moving toward the electrode), whereas

the right precordial leads (V1) have a deep negative wave (the delay is moving away from the electrode). Since normal left to right septal activation does not occur in LBBB, the normal septal q wave in lead V6 is lost. Furthermore, because the QRS from the left ventricle is delayed in LBBB, the left side of the LV QRS fuses with the QRS of the right ventricle, masking the Q wave. Often, this produces a notch in the LBBB R wave in lead V6, which may also be seen. Also note prominent repolarization abnormalities (ST-T changes in lead V6).

Figure 2-6. Right bundle branch block. Note the wide "M-shaped" QRS complex in lead V1. V1 typically is triphasic (rSR′ pattern) with the initial r of lesser amplitude than the subsequent R. V6 has a terminal S that is widened and of less amplitude than the initial R.

Figure 2-7. Left bundle branch block. Note the wide QRS complex and absence of a q wave in leads I and V6. V1 has a small r and a deep S with a rapid downslope. A broad, slurred monophasic R wave is present in lead V6 (and a notch in V5). In LBBB there is a broad, usually notched "M-shaped" R (the notch indicating the 2 asynchronous R waves, one from the right ventricle and the later one from the left ventricle) in leads I, V5–V6, and aVL. Because of abnormal septal depolarization, there is a marked loss of initial R wave voltage in precordial leads V1-V3, and absence of a small q wave normally seen in V6.

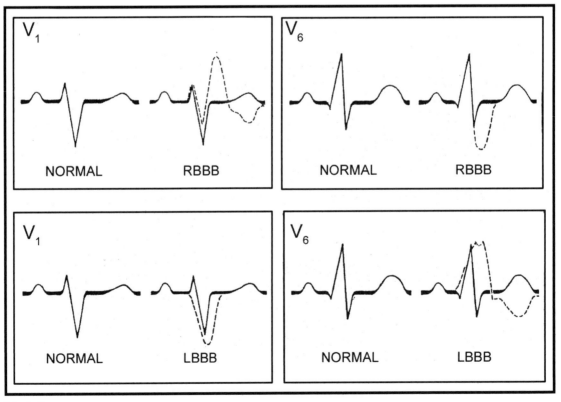

Fig. 2-5.

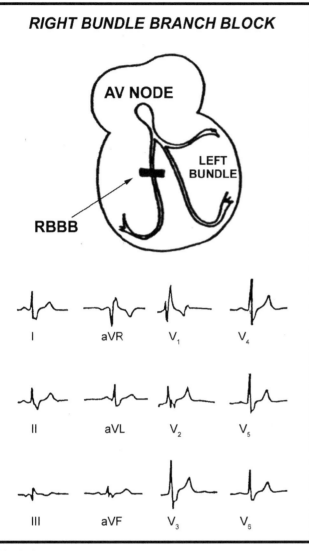

RIGHT BUNDLE BRANCH BLOCK

AV NODE

LEFT BUNDLE

RBBB

I aVR V₁ V₄

II aVL V₂ V₅

III aVF V₃ V₆

Fig. 2-6.

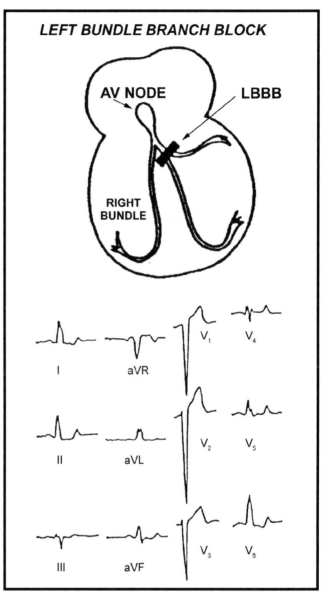

LEFT BUNDLE BRANCH BLOCK

AV NODE LBBB

RIGHT BUNDLE

I aVR V₁ V₄

II aVL V₂ V₅

III aVF V₃ V₆

Fig. 2-7.

The QRS may also be prolonged in other cases where there is aberrant conduction through ventricular myocardial tissue. For instance, a ventricular contraction resulting from an abnormal ectopic discharging focus in the ventricle, such as a premature ventricular contraction (PVC), characteristically results in a widened QRS of abnormal shape (see **Chapter 5**).

The *QRS width (interval)* can also be increased (0.12 seconds or more) in ventricular hypertrophy (because it takes longer to depolarize the abnormally thick muscle), ventricular pre-excitation (due to abnormal activation of the ventricle), and severe hyperkalemia (often the result of renal failure or certain medications, e.g., angiotensin converting enzyme [ACE] inhibitors).

The QRS *height* should be measured for possible ventricular hypertrophy. The normal QRS complex in the precordial leads is less than 25 mm high. Increased

QRS amplitude (high voltage) may be a normal finding in young, athletic, or thin individuals. *Left ventricular hypertrophy* is suggested with an S wave in V1 + R wave in V5 or V6 ≥ 35 mm, or R wave in aVL >11 mm in height. *Right ventricular hypertrophy* is suggested with an R wave height >S wave in V1, with an R wave in V1 >7 mm, with the R wave becoming progressively smaller on proceeding from V1 to V6, along with right axis deviation (see below under *QRS Axis*).

Figure 2-8. Left ventricular hypertrophy (**top**) resulting in a tall R wave in lead V6 and a deep S wave in lead V1. When the sum of the S wave in V1 and the R wave in V5 or V6 is >35 mm in the age group over 35 years, a voltage criterion for LV hypertrophy is present. In addition to voltage, changes suggesting

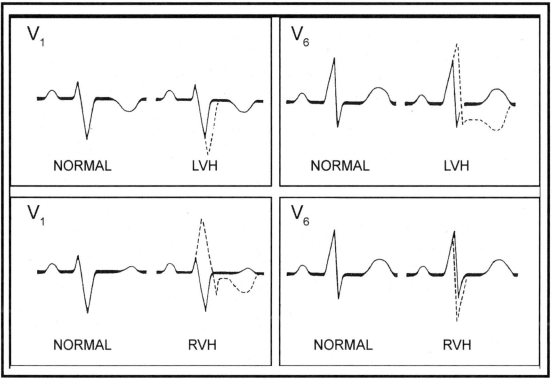

Fig. 2-8.

LV hypertrophy include left axis deviation (**Figure 2-13**), prolongation of the QRS interval, along with ST segment depression and T wave inversion (as seen in lead V6), which suggests LV *strain* (so-called *hockey stick* appearance of the QRS-ST-T complex) (**Figure 2-11F**). Large P waves due to left atrial enlargement may also be present.

Right ventricular hypertrophy (**bottom**). Since the right ventricle is to the right of and anterior to the left ventricle, right ventricular hypertrophy results in increased anterior forces (tall R waves) in the right precordial leads (V1) and a deep S wave in lead V6. The R/S ratio in lead V1 is >1, and the R/S ratio in lead V6 is <1. Right axis deviation (**Figure 2-13**) along with ST segment depression and T wave inversion in the right precordial leads (V1) suggests RV strain. Tall, peaked P waves due to right atrial enlargement may also be present.

Worthy of mention, the ECG cannot be used to reliably diagnose ventricular hypertrophy in the presence of bundle branch block, ventricular pre-excitation (WPW syndrome), paced ventricular rhythm, or ventricular arrhythmias.

The QRS should be assessed for the presence of normal or abnormal Q waves. A normal q wave should have a width of ≤0.04 seconds and a height <25% that of the QRS complex. While small negative initial deflections (q waves) are normal, large Q waves can be due to an electrically unexcitable area just under the recording electrode and frequently indicate a past MI.

Low voltage QRS complexes (< 5 mm in limb leads and/or < 10 mm in precordial leads) are commonly present in COPD, obesity, hypothyroidism, and pericardial effusion (due to air, fat, or fluid, respectively, between the heart and chest wall), and extensive MI, myocardial fibrosis, or infiltrative cardiomyopathy, e.g., amyloid (due to scarring, infiltration, or replacement of the myocardium).

Normally, the R wave becomes progressively taller as one progresses from V1 to V6 (**Figure 1-7**). A number of conditions, however, may be associated with "poor R wave progression" in leads V1 to V3–V4. These conditions include LV hypertrophy, RV hypertrophy, chronic pulmonary disease, anteroseptal MI, conduction defects (e.g., LBBB), left anterior hemiblock (blockage of the left anterior fascicle of the conduction system), cardiomyopathy, chest wall deformity, normal variant, and lead misplacement. Incorrect lead placement can lead to misdiagnosis and makes comparisons with previous ECGs difficult.

The T Wave

The T wave represents repolarization of the ventricles. T waves are normally upright in all ECG leads except aVR and V1, where they are typically inverted. Many factors can influence the T wave (e.g., metabolic disturbances, drug effect, autonomic stimuli, myocardial hypertrophy, bundle branch block, ischemia, or inflammation). If you suspect that the T wave is abnormally tall, consider hyperkalemia or an acute coronary syndrome (in the appropriate clinical context). Keep in mind, however, that tall T waves are often just a variant of normal.

Figure 2-9. Electrolyte imbalances affecting the T wave. Alterations in the serum electrolytes can produce dramatic changes in the ECG because of their roles in membrane repolarization and depolarization. As you will recall, influx and efflux of these ions across cell membranes are the basis for the electrical activity of cells.

Hyperkalemia causes peaked T waves along with flattened P waves and a widened QRS complex. If severe, the QRS complexes and T waves merge to form a *sine wave pattern*. Hypokalemia may produce flat T waves and prominent U waves (see below). Note the short QT interval in hypercalcemia, and prolonged QT interval in hypocalcemia.

The U Wave

A U wave, which follows the T wave, indicates poorly understood ventricular afterpotentials. Lead II and a slow heart rate provide the best opportunity to observe a U wave in the normal ECG tracing. In addition to bradycardia, *positive* U waves may occur with central nervous system disease, antiarrhythmic medication, and electrolyte disturbances (e.g., hypokalemia, hypomagnesemia). Causes of a *negative* U wave include LV hypertrophy and ischemia.

The PR Interval

The PR interval, QRS duration, and QT interval are measured from the limb leads (I, II, III, aVR, aVL, aVF).

The PR interval (normally 0.12–0.20 seconds) can be shorter than normal if the impulse originates in an ectopic site close to or in the AV junction (*junctional rhythm*) and in preexcitation syndromes, where the electrical impulse is conducted faster than normal through an accessory pathway that bypasses the AV node and bundle of His.

The PR interval may be longer than normal if the electrical impulse is abnormally delayed traveling through the AV node (e.g., first-degree AV block, see **Figure 5-22**). Common causes of first-degree AV block include normal variant, athletic conditioning, high vagal tone, medications (e.g., digitalis, beta blockers, rate-slowing calcium channel blockers [e.g., verapamil, diltiazem], and certain antiarrhythmic agents [e.g., amiodarone]), and a diseased AV node.

Although the normal PR segment is flat (isoelectric), it can be elevated or depressed in atrial ischemia or infarction, respectively. Pericarditis is also associated with PR segment depression, reflecting abnormal atrial repolarization related to atrial epicardial inflammation.

The ST Segment

While the *ST segment*, like the PR segment, is usually flat and at the baseline (isoelectric), small deviations are not always pathological (e.g., non-specific ST changes). As part of a complete ECG interpretation, the ST segment is assessed for deviations.

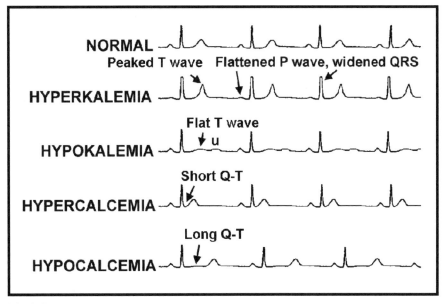

Fig. 2-9.

Figure 2-10. The normal ST segment and its variations in early repolarization, ischemia and infarction. Note the ST segment is normally isoelectric (flat, at the baseline) from the J point (junction of the QRS complex and the ST segment) until it gradually slopes into the shoulder of the T wave. Many healthy young individuals have slightly elevated concave upward ST segments (like a "smile"), particularly in the precordial leads (so-called *early repolarization*). During spontaneous angina pectoris or an exercise stress test, the ST segment is horizontal and depressed (*ischemic pattern*). When ischemia progresses to a transmural MI, convex ST segment elevation (like a "frown") occurs (*injury pattern*).

Although convex upward ("domed") ST elevation is usually the earliest change noted in acute MI due to prolonged coronary artery occlusion, it is not pathognomonic. It may be seen in other forms of myocardial injury, including *Takotsubo (stress) cardiomyopathy*, cocaine use, and *variant (Prinzmetal's) angina* (from coronary artery vasospasm), and as a stable change with *ventricular aneurysm* (persisting for months to years after an acute MI). In *pericarditis*, the elevated ST segment tends to be concave upward, but can easily be differentiated from acute ST segment elevation MI by its presence throughout all of the leads (except aVR, V1). (See **Figure 2-11D.**) As mentioned, sometimes the ST segment may be slightly elevated above the baseline in perfectly healthy people as a normal variant (i.e.,

early repolarization pattern), especially in young males, and closely resembles the concave upward ST elevation pattern of acute pericarditis.

Reciprocal ST depression in opposite ECG leads is highly characteristic of acute MI.

Figure 2-11. ST and T waves configurations in a variety of cardiac disease states and noncardiac conditions.

A. Hyperacute peaked T wave in early acute MI. Upsloping ST segment depression followed by hyperacute peaked T waves (so-called *de Winter's sign*) may also be seen in acute MI.

B. Typical convex upward ST segment elevation, along with Q wave and inversion of the T wave (see **Chapter 3**) in acute MI. If ST segment elevation persists, it may be a clue to LV aneurysm formation.

C. T wave inversion in myocardial ischemia or non-ST elevation (non Q wave) MI. *Subendocardial infarction* is a type of non Q wave infarction in which the infarct involves only the subendocardial part of the myocardium (which lies near the ventricular cavity), rather than the full thickness of the myocardium. The subendocardial region is the most susceptible part of the myocardium to infarct. In this type of non Q wave MI, the ST segment is depressed, rather than elevated. ST depression also occurs in ischemia (short of

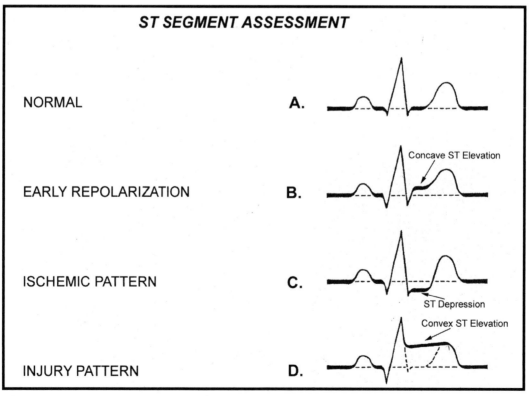

Fig. 2-10.

infarction) as in an abnormal stress test (see **G**). Deep T wave inversions in precordial leads V1-V4 may be seen with high-grade LAD stenosis (so-called *Wellen's pattern*). Of note, giant T wave inversions (so-called *cerebral T waves*) may also be seen in central nervous system diseases (see **Figure 3-22**).

D. Concave upward ST segment elevation along with PR segment depression in acute pericarditis.
E. Concave upward ST segment and J point elevation in early repolarization.
F. Downsloping ST segment merging into T wave inversion (so-called *strain pattern*) in LV hypertrophy.
G. Horizontal ST segment depression in myocardial ischemia, or non-ST elevation (non Q wave) MI or subendocardial infarction (see **C**).
H. Transient ST segment elevation in variant or Prinzmetal's angina and Takotsubo (*stress*) cardiomyopathy.
I. Horizontal ST segment depression and low voltage with non-specific ST-T changes often seen in coronary artery disease (CAD).
J. Scooped or downward coving (valley-like) ST segment seen with digitalis effect (**Mnemonic:** "Dig a valley.")
K. Coved ST segment elevation and RBBB morphology in *Brugada syndrome*.
L. J or Osborn wave simulating ST segment elevation in hypothermia (*camel-hump sign*).

Although ST depression is most often associated with myocardial ischemia, other common causes include LV and RV hypertrophy, dilated and hypertrophic cardiomyopathies, LBBB, RBBB, hypokalemia, and certain medications, e.g., digitalis, which causes a characteristic sagging (scooped-out) appearance (**Figure 2-11J**). In addition, many individuals have resting ECG tracings with minor degrees of ST depression and/or T wave changes, which in the absence of other objective findings, should not lead you to the mistaken diagnosis of heart disease.

ST-T WAVE ABNORMALITIES

A HYPERACUTE PEAKED T WAVE IN EARLY ACUTE MI

B CONVEX ST ELEVATION IN ACUTE MI

C T WAVE INVERSION IN MYOCARDIAL ISCHEMIA

D CONCAVE ST ELEVATION IN ACUTE PERICARDITIS

E CONCAVE ST ELEVATION IN EARLY REPOLARIZATION

F LV HYPERTROPHY WITH "STRAIN"

G HORIZONTAL ST DEPRESSION IN MYOCARDIAL ISCHEMIA

H TRANSIENT ST ELEVATION IN PRINZMETAL'S ANGINA

I NON SPECIFIC ST-T CHANGES

J DIGITALIS EFFECT

K COVED ST ELEVATION IN BRUGADA SYNDROME

L J (OSBORN) WAVE IN HYPOTHERMIA

Fig. 2-11.

The QT Interval

The QT interval varies normally with heart rate (the faster the heart rate, the shorter the QT). It is measured from the start of the QRS to the end of the T wave. The corrected interval is obtained by dividing the measured QT interval in seconds by the square root of the R-R interval in seconds (so-called *Bazett's formula*). The normal corrected QT interval is 0.44 seconds (in men) and 0.46 seconds (in women). A quick determination can be done if the heart rate is between 60 and 100 beats per minute by noting that the normal QT interval in that setting should measure less than one half of the R-R interval. If the QT interval is more than one half of the R-R interval, it is prolonged. With faster rates it may become slightly longer than half of the R-R interval, but this "rule of thumb" is sufficient for most purposes.

A long QT interval can be congenital (e.g., *Romano-Ward syndrome*, *Jervell and Lange-Nielsen syndrome*). A long QT interval may also be acquired as a result of

- Antiarrhythmic drugs (e.g., quinidine, disopyramide, procainamide, amiodarone, sotalol, and dofetilide)
- Macrolide antibiotics (e.g., erythromycin)
- Psychotropic drugs (e.g., tricyclic antidepressants, phenothiazines)
- Electrolyte disturbances (e.g., hypokalemia, hypomagnesemia)
- Central nervous system diseases (e.g., subarachnoid hemorrhage)

It may predispose an individual to the development of a specific type of polymorphic VT called *torsades de pointes* (twisting of the points) (see **Figure 2-12**).

Figure 2-12. ECG manifestations of the *long QT syndrome* (LQTS). In LQTS, the time it takes the heart muscle to recharge (the QT interval) is prolonged (usually >0.44 sec), leaving the individual susceptible to an unstable, dangerously rapid heart rhythm referred to as *polymorphic ventricular tachycardia* (*torsades de pointes*).

QRS Axis

The QRS axis represents the major vector direction of electrical activity (depolarization) in the ventricles. It is determined by analyzing the deflections of the QRS complexes in the limb leads. A 360° axial array, called the hexaxial reference system, combines all six limb leads in the frontal plane into one picture so that the QRS axis may be determined.

Figure 2-13. Left. The QRS axis is illustrated as a circular schematic called the *hexaxial reference system*. Using the positive or negative deflections of the QRS complex in both leads I and II is a simple method for approximating the axis. Some references recommend using leads I and aVF (rather than leads I and II) to determine whether the mean QRS axis is within the normal range (-30° to +90°) However, using leads I and aVF can erroneously classify a mean QRS axis between 0° and -30° as "abnormal."

Right. The mean QRS axis (the overall direction of the wave of myocardial cell depolarization passing through the myocardium) normally falls between -30° and 90°. An analysis of the direction of the QRS complexes in leads I and II may provide the information for a qualitative assessment of the axis. If the complexes in leads I and II are both predominantly positive, the axis is normal. If the complex is negative in lead I and positive in lead II, right axis deviation is present.

(**Mnemonic:** Visualize the numbers I and II written on the patient's chest so that I is on the patient's right side and II is on the patient's left. In right axis deviation, I, on the right, is negative; in left axis deviation, II, on the left, is negative.) If the complex is positive in lead I and negative in lead II, left axis deviation is present; and if the complex is negative in both leads I and II, extreme axis deviation is present. If the QRS complex is equiphasic (positive and negative deflections are equal) in all six limb leads, the axis is said to be indeterminate. (Try to keep in mind **Figure 2-13** for easy recall of these criteria.)

The QRS axis can give a clue to many different pathologic states. *Left axis deviation* can occur in LV hypertrophy, inferior wall MI (MI on the diaphragmatic surface of the heart often including the right ventricle), and left anterior fascicular block (conduction block in the anterior division of the left bundle, which produces

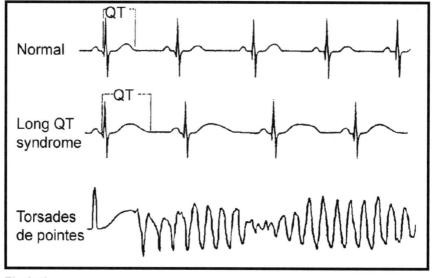

Fig. 2-12.

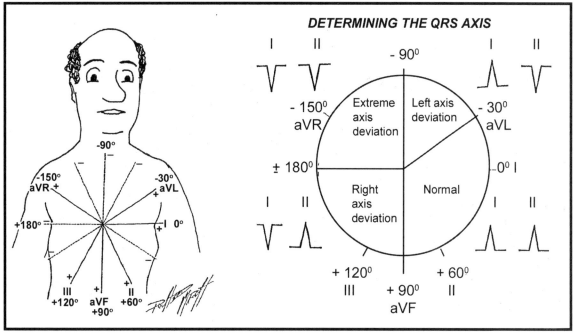

Fig. 2-13.

unopposed, delayed depolarization upward and to the left of the anterior portion of the left ventricle).

Right axis deviation can occur in RV hypertrophy, acute right heart strain (massive pulmonary embolism), left posterior fascicular block (conduction block in the posterior division of the left bundle, which produces unopposed, delayed depolarization downward and to the right of the posterior portion of the left ventricle), lateral wall MI, and left and right arm lead reversal (look for an inverted P wave in lead I). The axis tends to point toward ventricular hypertrophy and away from infarction.

Deviation of the electrical axis in the presence of BBB (particularly RBBB) is often a clue to more extensive disease of the conduction system (e.g., block of the left anterior or posterior fascicle in addition to RBBB, which is termed *bifascicular block*).

Figure 2-14 summarizes a systematic approach to ECG interpretation. Once the essentials of ECG interpretation are understood and practiced in a repetitive manner, your ability to read and interpret ECGs will improve significantly. In the chapters that follow, we will turn our attention to the major cardiac and noncardiac conditions encountered in clinical practice that can cause the abnormalities seen on the 12-lead ECG.

FIGURE 2-14
SYSTEMATIC APPROACH TO ECG INTERPRETATION

Basic Concepts
• Observe name and date (checking to be sure it is the correct patient's ECG).
• Assess age and gender.
• Check for technical quality of ECG and other factors (e.g., voltage calibration of the ECG machine).
• Compare with patient's previous ECGs.

Determine Cardiac Rhythm
• Is the rhythm regular or irregular?
• Identify atrial activity (P waves) and ventricular activity (QRS complexes).
• Determine the P-QRS relationship.

Measure Heart Rate
• Use the following methods.
  —Counting method (300–150–100–75–60–50)
  —Number of beats in 6 seconds x 10
• Is the rate normal (60–100 bpm), bradycardia (<60 bpm), or tachycardia (>100 bpm)?

Evaluate P Wave Morphology
• Inspect P wave in leads II and V1 for right and left atrial enlargement. What are the amplitude, duration and direction?

Assess PR, QRS, and QT Intervals
• PR interval–Is it normal (0.12–0.20 sec.), short or prolonged?
• QRS interval–Is it normal (≤0.10 sec) or abnormal? If ≥ 0.12 sec, check the QRS for bundle branch block.
• QT interval–What is the duration? Normal QT ≤ one-half of the R-R interval, (if heart rate is normal).

Determine Mean QRS Axis (in the limb leads)
• Is it normal (+90° to –30°), left axis deviation, or right axis deviation?
• Also assess R wave progression in the precordial leads. Is it normal, poor progression, or early transition?

Evaluate QRS Complex, ST and T Wave Morphologies
• Is a Q wave present or absent? If pathologic Q waves present, check the anatomic distribution: septal leads (V1, V2), anterior leads (V3, V4), lateral leads (I, aVL, V5, V6), and inferior leads (II, III, aVF). Q waves normal width <0.04 seconds; height <25% of QRS complex.
• Is the QRS amplitude normal, increased, or decreased? Check for left or right ventricular hypertrophy.
• Is the ST segment elevated, depressed or isoelectric? Check for ischemia, infarction, pericarditis, metabolic and/or chemical abnormalities.
• Is the T wave upright or inverted?
• Is the amplitude increased or diminished?

Identify Abnormal ECG Patterns
• Myocardial ischemia and infarction
• Cardiac chamber enlargement and hypertrophy
• Arrhythmias and conduction disturbances
• Miscellaneous patterns (e.g., pericarditis, WPW syndrome, electrolyte imbalances, drug effects)
• Is a pacemaker present? If so, is it pacing, capturing, and sensing appropriately?

Part II. Major ECG Abnormalities: Diagnostic Clues And Clinical Correlations

A wide variety of clinical conditions, both cardiac and noncardiac, can cause abnormalities on the 12-lead ECG. When you first encounter a patient suspected to have a cardiac problem, you do not know what pertinent ECG findings may be present that will provide a clue that leads to or perhaps makes the diagnosis.

Some abnormalities (e.g., cardiac arrhythmias and conduction disturbances) are determined *only* by the ECG. Others (e.g., myocardial ischemia and infarction) can be diagnosed or clarified when placed in the appropriate clinical context. Still others (e.g., pericarditis) can be suggested when a specific ECG pattern is observed.

The accuracy of ECG interpretation is greatly improved when clinical information (e.g., the patient's age, gender, presenting symptoms, and list of medications) is considered. Any ECG abnormalities detected can then be interpreted in relation to the other aspects of the patient's evaluation. A prior ECG for comparison is also extremely helpful (particularly in patients with chest pain and abnormal ST segments) and should be sought whenever possible.

The following chapters will present a practical clinical overview of the major ECG abnormalities encountered in clinical practice along with their diagnostic clues and clinical correlations.

3

Myocardial Ischemia And Infarction

Myocardial ischemia is due to insufficient oxygen supply to the ventricular muscle. It may be transient, causing the coronary syndromes *stable* (exertional) and *unstable* (rest) *angina*, or more severe and prolonged, causing death of a portion of heart muscle, called *myocardial infarction*. Chronic stable angina is caused by a fixed, flow limiting atherosclerotic plaque in the coronary artery that fails to meet the heart's demand for oxygen (supply-demand ischemic mismatch). Most acute coronary syndromes result from a plaque rupture and thrombus that partially occludes (unstable angina) or totally occludes (myocardial infarction) the coronary artery and impairs blood flow. The standard 12-lead ECG, despite its limitations, is a highly useful clinical tool in evaluating patients with chest pain of suspected ischemic etiology.

Figure 3-1. Patterns of ECG abnormalities during ischemia. Ischemia denotes temporary, reversible reduction of blood supply with deprivation of oxygen to the heart muscle. Myocardial ischemia primarily affects repolarization of the ventricle and is present when 1 mm or more horizontal or downsloping ST segment depression occurs. Transient (horizontal or downsloping) ST segment *depression* during an episode of chest pain suggestive of classic angina, provides a clue to myocardial ischemia due to fixed obstructive CAD (where there is a fixed narrowing of the vessel lumen). Transient symmetrically shaped T wave *inversion* is also a sign of myocardial ischemia. Transient ST segment *elevation*, though, suggests variant or Prinzmetal's angina and provides a clue to underlying coronary artery spasm.

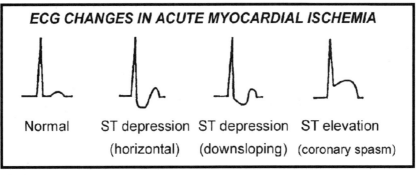

Fig. 3-1.

Classic (Stable and Unstable) Angina Pectoris

Figure 3-2. ECG findings during an episode of angina pectoris. **Left.** Note middle-aged male clutching his chest (Levine's sign) with beads of perspiration on his forehead. **Right.** Classic angina is thought to be due to transient subendocardial ischemia. The ECG taken during the ischemic episode reveals transient ST segment depression that resolves once the chest pain subsides.

Prinzmetal's (Variant) Angina

Figure 3-3A. Spasm of the left anterior descending coronary artery in a patient with variant (Prinzmetal's) angina. Both the typical ST segment elevation and chest pain resolve after relief of coronary vasospasm by nitroglycerin.

Figure 3-3B. ECG tracing from a young female with migraine headaches and variant (Prinzmetal's) angina. At the onset of chest pain, there is marked ST segment elevation in lead II (due to spasm of the right coronary artery). Note that as the pain subsides several minutes later, ST segment elevation returns to baseline and the ECG is normal.

Ischemia causes complex changes in the electrophysiologic properties of the myocardial cells. These changes produce a voltage gradient (flow of current) between nonischemic and ischemic cells, resulting in deviations of the ST segment and T waves during transient episodes of myocardial ischemia. When ischemia is more severe and prolonged,

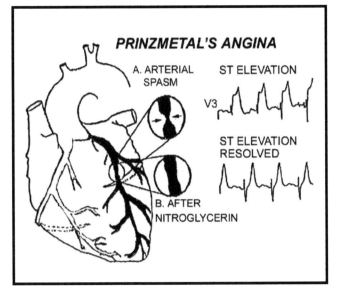

Fig. 3-3A.

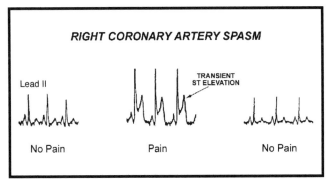

Fig. 3-3B.

myocardial injury or infarction (necrosis) can result (see below). Profound ST segment elevation or depression in multiple leads usually indicates very severe ischemia affecting large regions of the myocardium. These ECG abnormalities can be minimized or aborted by restoring blood flow to the myocardium (reperfusion). It is important to realize, however, that the resting ECG may be entirely normal between episodes of angina pectoris (i.e., when no symptoms and no ischemia are present) in 50% of patients with significant CAD without a history of previous MI. Furthermore, some episodes of transient myocardial ischemia, particularly those associated with disease in the left circumflex coronary artery, do not lead to overt abnormalities on the ECG.

ST Elevation (Q wave) MI

With *injury*, which in cardiology refers to (early) infarction, there is prolonged (but potentially

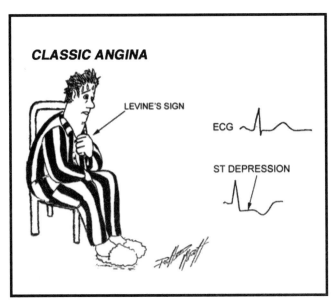

Fig. 3-2.

reversible) reduction in blood supply to the myocardium along with ST segment elevation. The ST segment elevation that appears in the ECG leads overlying the infarcted myocardium is believed to result from injured myocardial cells adjacent to the infarcted zone that produce abnormal electrical currents. These electrical currents may result, in part, from premature repolarization of the injured myocardial cells, making their surface charge electrically positive relative to the neighboring normal cells. When acute severe ischemia is transmural (or nearly so), the overall ST vector (current of injury) is shifted in the direction of the electropositive outer (epicardial) ventricular layer, resulting in ST segment elevation in the leads that overlie the area of infarction. Reciprocal ST segment depression will occur in the ECG leads oriented opposite the location of infarction. Although there are electrophysiologic explanations as to why these ST segment changes occur, it is simply easier to remember the specific ECG patterns in the particular leads of the various kinds of infarction than to go through the logic of trying to figure them out from the mechanisms.

Q waves are a sign of (late) *infarction*, i.e., irreversible death of heart muscle due to prolonged coronary artery occlusion caused by an acute thrombus superimposed on a ruptured atherosclerotic plaque. In time, the ST elevation may disappear, but the Q wave remains as an indicator of previous MI (**Figure 3-4**).

Figure 3-4. *Acute MI* characteristically produces a sequence of changes in the ECG that involve both the QRS and the ST-T complexes. This figure depicts ECG evolution in acute ST elevation (Q wave) myocardial infarction (STEMI). The "classic" ECG changes of acute MI begins with hyperacute upright T waves, followed by ST segment elevation (current of injury pattern) in the leads reflecting the site of infarction. Note that the ST segment elevation (convex upward, domed) occurs prior to the formation of the Q wave. During these early hours, percutaneous coronary intervention (PCI)/thrombolysis is often undertaken to reverse the process. As time passes, the Q wave forms, the ST segment becomes less elevated, and the T wave inversion reverts to upright again. The Q waves that appear during the course of an MI are related to the necrotic myocardium (scar), which is electrically inactive. Since the infarcted area does not generate electrical forces, the surface electrode overlying this area "sees" only the negative portion of the depolarization wave of the opposite wall, which is now unopposed, and a negative deflection or pathologic Q wave results. The final outcome of what the ECG looks like varies greatly, depending on the amount of myocardial damage. Q waves usually persist indefinitely, but may disappear over weeks to months. If successful early reperfusion is achieved, the elevated ST segment returns to baseline without subsequent T wave inversion or Q wave formation.

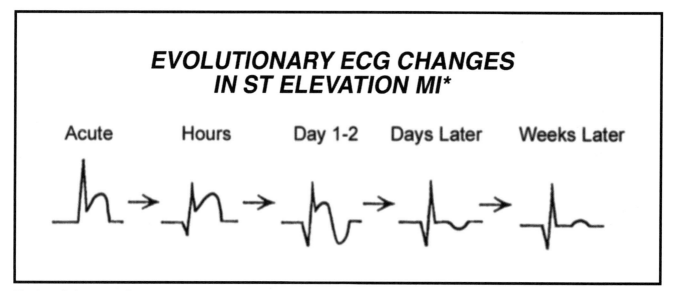

EVOLUTIONARY ECG CHANGES IN ST ELEVATION MI*

Acute   Hours   Day 1-2   Days Later   Weeks Later

Fig. 3-4. (*also termed acute Q wave MI)

Non-ST Elevation (non-Q Wave) MI

Figure 3-5. Schematic representation of a non-ST segment elevation myocardial infarction (non-STEMI) as recorded in a lead overlying the left ventricle at that location. Non-ST segment elevation MIs (non Q wave MIs) represent incomplete infarcts that selectively affect the subendocardial part of the myocardium. The flow of current from the normally perfused myocardial cells in the outer layer of the heart (epicardium) toward the electropositive ischemic cells in the inner layer (subendocardium) moves away from the ECG leads overlying the infarcted region, resulting in ST segment depression. Non-STEMIs also cause T wave inversion, although they can manifest ST segment depression alone.

To summarize: In a patient presenting with chest pain compatible with an *acute coronary syndrome* (ACS), an umbrella term that includes unstable angina, non-STEMI, and STEMI, ECG evidence of tall positive (hyperacute) T waves and ST segment elevation, as opposed to ST segment depression and T wave inversion, helps differentiate STEMI from unstable angina and non-STEMI. Some patients with an acute MI present with upsloping ST segment depression followed by tall positive (hyperacute) T waves (so-called *de Winter's sign*). This should be treated as a STEMI equivalent, since typically it is caused by an acute coronary occlusion.

Localization of Myocardial Infarction

A basic knowledge of the coronary anatomy is an essential requisite to understanding and interpreting the ECG changes of myocardial infarction.

Figure 3-6. The coronary arteries. Note that the left main coronary artery bifurcates into the left anterior descending (LAD) and left circumflex coronary arteries.

- The LAD provides blood supply to the anterior wall and interventricular septum, and the left circumflex to the lateral wall.
- The right coronary artery (RCA) provides blood to the inferior (diaphragmatic) wall of the left and/or right ventricle, the sinus node in 55% and AV node in 90% of cases. (At other times the left circumflex artery supplies the SA or AV node.) Sudden total occlusion of the RCA results in an acute inferior MI (leads II, III, aVF) and/or right ventricular (RV) MI (right-sided ECG lead V4R). Sinus bradycardia (from SA nodal involvement) and first-, second-, or third-degree heart block (from AV nodal involvement) may occur (see **Figure 5-22**).
- Sudden occlusion of the left main coronary artery leads to extensive anterior MI (leads V1–V6, I, aVL), pump failure, and sudden death. ST elevation in lead aVR greater than in lead V1 may be a useful clue.
- Sudden occlusion of the LAD coronary artery leads to anterior MI (leads V1–V6) with LV failure, atrial and ventricular arrhythmias, bundle branch block and Mobitz type II (fixed PR interval with abrupt dropped beat; see **Figure 5-22**) second-degree AV block due to involvement of the conduction system in the interventricular septum.

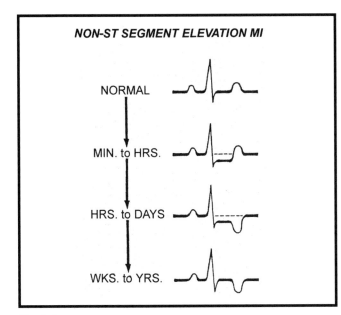

Fig. 3-5.

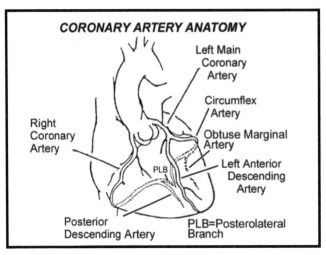

Fig. 3-6.

- Sudden occlusion of the left circumflex coronary artery leads to acute lateral MI (leads I, aVL). In ~10-20% of patients, this artery (rather than the RCA) also supplies the inferior and posterior walls of the LV. The standard 12-lead ECG does not have electrodes to look at the posterior surface of the LV (or RV). Posterior MI is manifest reciprocally (tall R waves with ST depression) in leads V1-V3 (*mirror image*). Posterior chest leads (V7-V9) help confirm the diagnosis.

Figure 3-7A. Schematic diagram showing the locations of myocardial infarctions. Although the right ventricle may become infarcted, infarction usually involves only the left ventricle.

ECG leads may be grouped according to the surfaces of the heart that they represent. ECG leads that "view" the same or adjacent areas of the heart are called *contiguous leads* (**Figure 3-7B**). The ECG taken during pain frequently identifies the specific area of infarct:

- *Anteroseptal* [V1-V4], with septal (V1-V2) and anterior (V3-V4)
- *Anterolateral* [V5-V6, I, AVL]
- *Lateral* [I, AVL]
- *Inferior* [II, III, AVF]
- *True posterior* (tall broad R waves with ST depression V1-V3--*mirror image*)

Figure 3-8 summarizes the areas of the heart affected by MI, and their corresponding arteries and ECG leads.

Pathologic Q waves develop in leads II, III, aVF (in inferior MI), I and aVL (in high lateral MI), V1-V4 (in anteroseptal MI), and an increase in R wave (reciprocal of the Q wave) in V1-V3 in true posterior MI. (See **Figures 3-9** through **3-12**.) A prominent R wave in V1, however, is not pathognomonic of true posterior MI, since similar changes are sometimes seen with RV hypertrophy, WPW syndrome, counterclockwise rotation of the heart, and RBBB.

LOCALIZATION OF MI

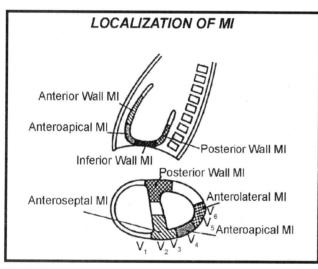

Anterior Wall MI
Anteroapical MI
Posterior Wall MI
Inferior Wall MI
Posterior Wall MI
Anteroseptal MI
Anterolateral MI
Anteroapical MI
V1 V2 V3 V4 V5 V6

Fig. 3-7A.

FIGURE 3-7B CONTIGUOUS ECG LEADS AND LOCATION OF MI			
Limb Leads		**Precordial Leads**	
I Lateral	aVR	V1 Septal	V4 Anterior
II Inferior	aVL Lateral	V2 Septal	V5 Lateral
III Inferior	aVF Inferior	V3 Anterior	V6 Lateral

Note: Posterior wall MI does not produce pathologic Q waves and ST elevation on the standard 12-lead ECG. It is diagnosed by visualizing reciprocal (mirror-image) changes, i.e., tall R waves and ST depression, in the anterior precordial leads (V1-V3)

FIGURE 3-8 ECG CLUES TO THE LOCATION OF MYOCARDIAL INFARCTION AND CORONARY ARTERY INVOLVED		
Location of Infarction	**ECG Leads**	**Coronary Artery**
Anterior		
• Extensive anterior	V1-V6, I, AVL	Left Main* Proximal LAD
• Anteroseptal	V1-V4	Left: LAD
• Anterolateral	V5-V6, I, AVL	Left: LAD
• Apical	V5, V6, I, II, AVF	Left: LAD (usual) Right: PDA
High lateral	I, AVL	Left: OMB of CFA Diagonal of LAD
Inferior (diaphragmatic)	II, III, AVF	Right: PDA (80%) Left CFA (20%)
Right ventricular	Right precordial leads e.g., V4R, V1-V2	Right: proximal
True posterior	Tall, broad R waves with ST depression V1-V3 (mirror image) Posterior chest leads e.g., V7-V9	Left: CFA Right: PL branch

LAD = left anterior descending; CFA = circumflex artery; PDA = posterior descending artery; OMB = obtuse marginal branch; PL = posterolateral branch
*Note: Widespread ST depression along with ST elevation in lead aVR >VI may be a useful clue to left main coronary artery occlusion.

Inferior Wall MI

Damage to the inferior (diaphragmatic) surface of the heart usually results from occlusion of the right coronary artery (or, less commonly, the left circumflex coronary artery). ECG changes can be seen in the inferior leads (II, III, and aVF) oriented over the area of damage. Reciprocal (mirror image) changes will be seen in the lateral leads (I and aVL) oriented opposite the area of infarction.

Figure 3-9. 12-lead ECG tracing in a patient with acute inferior MI. Note that the ST segment elevation in the inferior leads (II, III, and aVF) results in reciprocal ST segment depression in leads I and aVL.

Lateral Wall MI

Damage to the lateral wall of the heart results from occlusion of the left circumflex coronary artery. ECG changes will occur in the lateral leads I, aVL, V5 and V6. Reciprocal ECG changes may be seen in leads II, III, and aVF.

Figure 3-10. Acute lateral wall MI. Note the ST segment elevation in leads I and aVL, with reciprocal ST segment depression in the inferior leads II, III and AVF.

Anterior Wall MI

Damage to the anterior surface of the heart results from occlusion of the left anterior descending coronary artery. ECG changes are usually observed in the anterior leads (V1 through V4).

Figure 3-11. Anterior MI. Note the prominent Q waves with ST segment elevation and T wave inversion in leads V1–V4. Since ST segment elevation is also present in leads V5 and V6, the description "anterolateral wall MI" also applies.

Posterior Wall MI

Posterior wall MI may be seen in conjunction with inferior wall MI. It is usually caused by occlusion of the right or left circumflex coronary artery. Because there are no conventional ECG leads overlying the posterior wall of the heart, ECG evidence of infarction is inferred from reciprocal (mirror image) changes in the opposing anterior chest leads (V1-V3). These leads, which are oriented opposite the site of infarction, may reveal tall R waves, ST segment depression, and upright T waves.

Figure 3-12. Acute posterior MI. Q waves and ST elevation are represented reciprocally *(mirror images)* as tall R waves with ST segment depression in leads V1-V3. The inferior and/or lateral leads are often involved in the infarction process.

Evolution of Acute MI

Figures 3-13 through 3-15 show the characteristic evolutionary ECG changes that occur with anterior, posterior, and inferior wall MI. The various stages in the evolution of MI can usually be demonstrated in serial ECGs taken over a period of time.

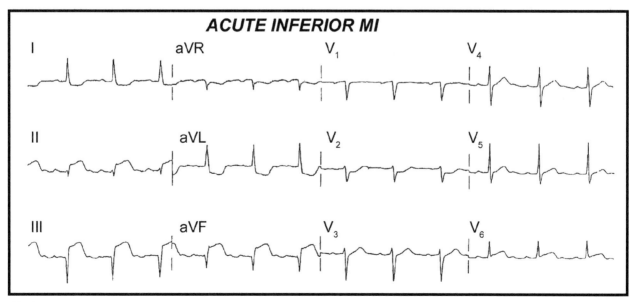

Fig. 3-9.

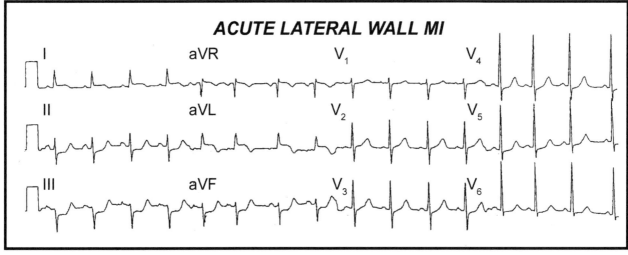

Fig. 3-10.

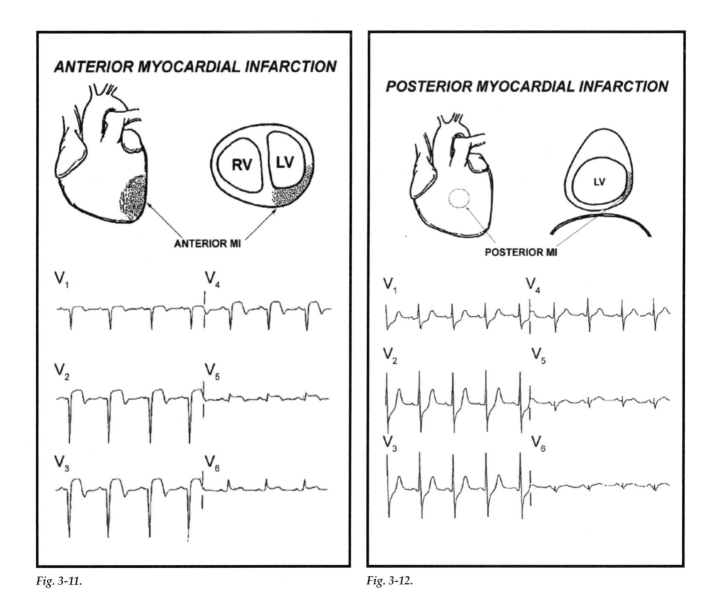

Fig. 3-11.

Fig. 3-12.

Figure 3-13. Typical evolutionary ECG changes of an *anterior wall MI* (seen through lead V1) compared with those of a *posterior wall MI* (seen through lead V1). The changes in the anterior wall MI are typical (as noted in **Figure 3-4**). However, since there are no posterior leads in a standard 12-lead ECG, a *posterior MI* is reflected by reciprocal changes in the anterior precordial leads that are the inverse *(mirror image)* of what one would see in leads overlying the posterior myocardium. Note the presence of ST segment depression (inverse of the current of injury) and a tall R wave (inverse of a Q wave) in lead V1.

Figure 3-14. Classic evolutionary ECG changes in acute *anterior MI*.

A. Hyperacute ST segment elevation and peaking of T waves.
B. Marked *(tombstone)* ST segment elevation in leads V1-V6, I and aVL. Multifocal premature ventricular contractions are also present.
C. Development of more pronounced Q waves and T wave inversion with regression of coved and convex upward (domed) ST segment elevation. Persistent ST segment elevation suggests LV aneurysm formation.

Figure 3-15. Classic evolutionary ECG changes in acute *inferior MI*.

A. Hyperacute ST segment elevation and peaking of T waves.
B. Marked *(tombstone)* ST segment elevation in leads II, III, aVF with "reciprocal" ST segment depression in precordial leads.
C. Loss of R waves, development of pathologic Q waves, T wave inversion and return of ST segment elevation toward baseline.

Right Ventricular MI

The right ventricle may also be involved in up to 40% of inferior wall MIs. The ECG changes of RV MI may be seen in precordial lead V1 or in unconventional right-sided chest leads.

ST segment elevation in lead III greater than in lead II is a useful clue to occlusion of the proximal right coronary artery. The occurrence of ST segment elevation and loss of R waves in right-sided chest leads (particularly V4R), in association with an inferior or posterior MI, are sensitive clinical clues to an *RV infarction*. (**Figure 3-16**).

Figure 3-16. Left. Location of right-sided precordial ECG leads (V1R-V6R).

Right. ECG tracing demonstrating acute *inferior wall MI* with *RV infarction*. Note ST segment elevation in leads II, III, aVF, along with ST segment elevation in leads V4R–V6R.

The 12-lead ECG remains the most important initial diagnostic tool in patients with acute MI. Combined

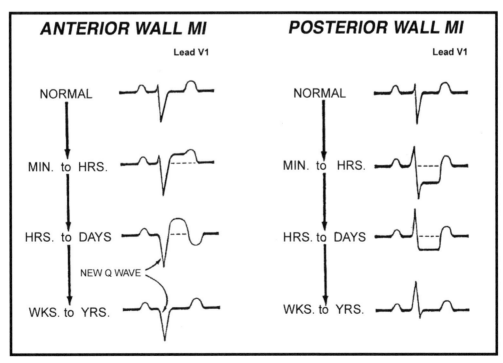

Fig. 3-13.

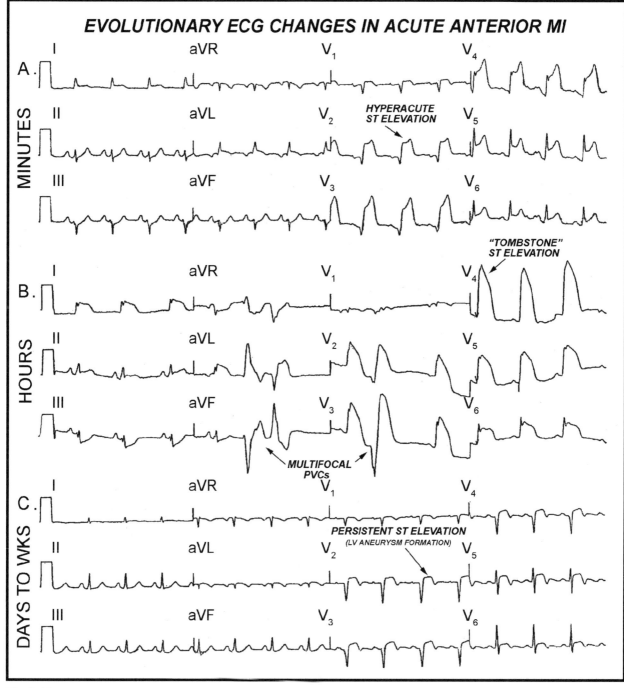

Fig. 3-14.

with the patient's history and physical examination, the 12-lead ECG is the major determinant of eligibility for PCI/thrombolysis. The two key ECG findings are ≥ 1 mm ST segment elevation (not disappearing rapidly as in Prinzmetal's angina) in two or more anatomically contiguous leads, or new (or presumably new) LBBB with specific ECG criteria (see below). Keep in mind that in patients who present with a presumed new anterior MI, ST segment elevation in V2-V3 ≥ 2 mm (in men) or ≥ 1.5 mm (in women) improves the diagnostic accuracy

ST Elevation MI in LBBB

Although patients presenting with an acute MI and new LBBB benefit significantly from rapid reperfusion therapy, a new LBBB, by itself, in a patient with chest pain is no longer considered a STEMI equivalent,

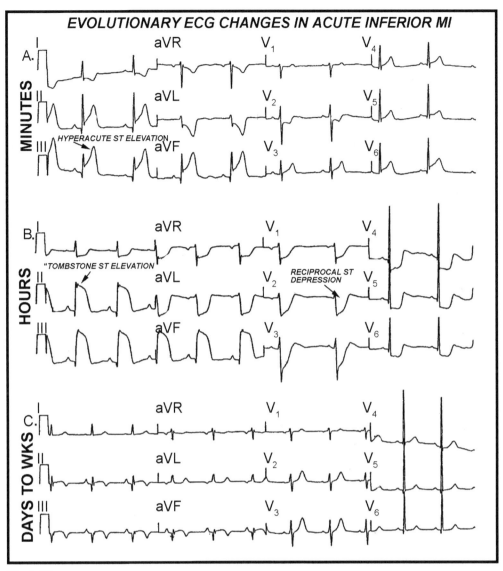

Fig. 3-15.

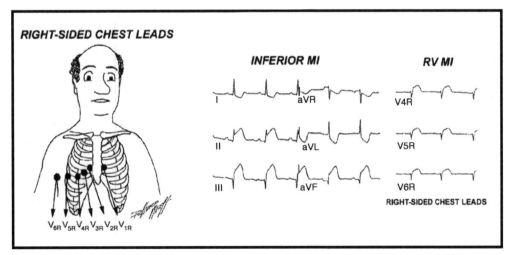

Fig. 3-16.

since only a minority of these patients are actually experiencing an acute MI. In patients with LBBB, ECG criteria that can more accurately diagnose an acute MI (with high specificity but poor sensitivity) include ST segment elevation ≥ 1 mm and concordant (in the same direction) with the QRS in any lead (strongest predictor), ST segment depression ≥ 1 mm and concordant with the QRS in leads V1 to V3, and ST segment elevation ≥ 5 mm and excessively discordant (in the opposite direction) with the QRS (weakest predictor), the so-called *Sgarbossa's criteria*. (See **Figure 3-17**.)

Figure 3-17. STEMI in left bundle branch block (LBBB) is strongly suggested by the presence of ST segment elevation that is ≥1 mm and concordant (in the same direction) with the QRS in leads V5 and V6, and ≥5 mm and excessively discordant (in the opposite direction) with the QRS in leads V2 and V3 (so-called *Sgarbossa's criteria*).

The Sgarbossa criteria used to assess for acute MI in the presence of LBBB may also be used in patients with ventricular paced rhythm (RV pacing demonstrates an LBBB pattern). Of note, the usual criteria used to diagnose acute MI may be used with RBBB since, unlike LBBB, it does not affect the initial portion of the QRS complex.

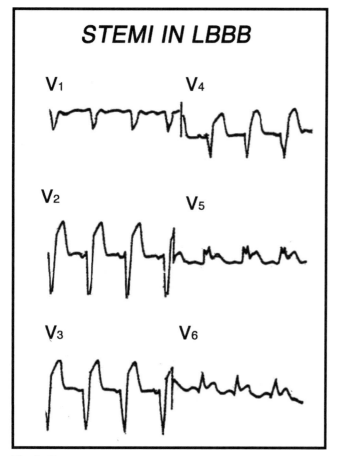

Fig. 3-17.

ECG Signs of Reperfusion

The ECG findings in the previous section suggest that the damage may involve recent thrombosis and that the patient may be a candidate for reperfusion therapy. No evidence of benefit from emergent reperfusion is found in patients with ischemic chest pain who lack either appropriate ST segment elevation or new LBBB with specific ECG criteria. Unlike patients with ST segment elevation MIs, those with non-ST segment elevation MIs (non Q wave MIs) do not benefit from thrombolytic therapy.

Figure 3-18. Clinical markers of reperfusion. **Left.** Serial ECG recording (leads V1-V3) in a patient with acute anterior MI treated with thrombolytic therapy. Note the ST segment elevation begins to decrease rapidly and falls by more than 50% over the next half hour. During this time, the patient reported rapid and complete relief of chest pain. Resolution of ST segment elevation is a good predictor of vessel patency. **Right.** The appearance of accelerated idioventricular rhythm (AIVR–a rhythm paced by a ventricular focus, rather than the SA node) often provides additional evidence of reperfusion.

In general, the larger the MI, the greater the mortality reduction with reperfusion therapy. The size of an MI is reflected by either the absolute number of leads showing ST segment elevation on the ECG, or a summation of the total ST segment deviations from the baseline (i.e., both ST segment depressions and elevations). Patients who present with ischemic chest pain and deep T wave inversions in multiple precordial leads (e.g., V1-V4), with or without cardiac enzyme elevations, typically have a high-grade stenosis in the proximal LAD coronary artery (so-called *Wellens pattern*). If untreated, these patients may go on to develop an extensive anterior MI within a few weeks to months

Limitations of the ECG in MI

While its clinical importance is beyond question, the ECG has many limitations. The initial ECG may remain normal for hours after an acute MI, and it may be diagnostic in only 50-60% of patients. Furthermore, although the presence of Q waves suggests prior MI, their absence is not helpful in excluding significant CAD. An MI may occur without diagnostic ECG changes (there may be only slight or even absent ST-T changes), depending on the extent, location, and associated ECG abnormalities (e.g., left bundle branch block, electronic ventricular pacemaker). In left ventricle infarct with LBBB, it is difficult to identify Q waves since the left ventricle depolarizes later than the right ventricle, and the Q wave part of the left ventricle QRS is buried within

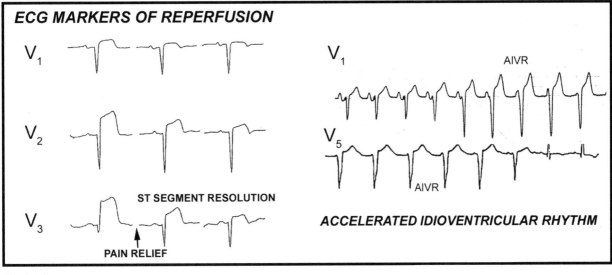

ECG MARKERS OF REPERFUSION

V₁

V₂

V₃

ST SEGMENT RESOLUTION

PAIN RELIEF

V₁

V₅

AIVR

AIVR

ACCELERATED IDIOVENTRICULAR RHYTHM

Fig. 3-18.

the preceding right ventricle depolarization. The ECG taken during the early stages of an acute MI, when the patient is most susceptible to primary ventricular fibrillation, may appear normal (in as many as 20% of cases). If the clinical suspicion is high, the normal ECG should not be considered evidence against the diagnosis. All too often a patient is sent home inappropriately from the emergency department with an acute MI because of an over-reliance on the ECG (**Figure 3-19**).

Figure 3-19. Lesson of the normal ECG. Note that leads V1–V3 from a 12-lead ECG taken in the Emergency Department in a patient who presented with chest pain were entirely normal. Fortunately, the patient was appropriately admitted to the coronary care unit based on the clinical history despite the normal ECG. Note that ST segment elevation and T wave peaking (so-called *hyperacute change*) appeared 2 hours later when chest pain intensified and clinical appearance worsened.

Despite sophisticated laboratory tests, including new cardiac serum markers (e.g., troponins) and imaging techniques, and the limitations cited above, the ECG still remains the most reliable and inexpensive tool for the rapid confirmation of acute MI, dictating appropriate triage and prompt treatment with life-saving reperfusion therapy.

Whenever possible, a prior ECG should be obtained to help determine if abnormalities seen on a current tracing are new or old. Without previous tracings, any ECG finding that cannot be proved to be old must be assumed to be new. On occasion, a new ECG abnormality can "erase" a previously existing one. Complete normalization of the ECG following a Q wave infarction is uncommon, but may occur particularly with smaller infarcts. Serial ECGs permit evaluation of the response to therapy and of progression, remission,

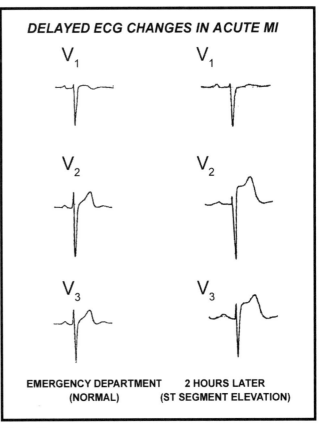

DELAYED ECG CHANGES IN ACUTE MI

V₁   V₁

V₂   V₂

V₃   V₃

EMERGENCY DEPARTMENT   2 HOURS LATER
(NORMAL)   (ST SEGMENT ELEVATION)

Fig. 3-19.

or persistence of an abnormality noted on the baseline tracing. For example, the ECG may be used to assess the response to a thrombolytic agent or to anti-ischemic therapy. Complete resolution of ST segment elevation promptly following thrombolytic therapy (or after PCI)

35

is a specific, although not sensitive, marker of successful reperfusion (**Figure 3-18**).

It is important not to over-interpret the ECG. A patient may have serious underlying heart disease with little or no abnormality on the ECG, or no detectable heart disease, but an abnormal ECG tracing. Reliance on computer-generated ECG interpretation can also result in potential mischief (i.e., incorrect, over- and/or under-diagnoses), occasionally with devastating clinical consequences. The computer analysis must be carefully reviewed and edited to avert misdiagnosis before a final interpretation is made. The range of normal is broad, and clinical circumstances should dictate the importance of a particular ECG observation. Examples:

- The presence of Q waves and a pseudo-"infarct" pattern on the ECG (e.g., in *Wolff-Parkinson White [WPW] syndrome*) does not always reflect CAD (**Figures 3-20** and **3-21**). The presence of delta waves helps distinguish WPW (see **Chapter 5**).

Figure 3-20. 12-lead ECG tracing in a patient with *WPW syndrome* simulating anteroseptal MI (due to delta waves distorting the QRS complexes in the anterior leads).

Figure 3-21. 12-lead ECG tracing in a patient with *WPW syndrome* mimicking inferior MI. This asymptomatic patient had a "routine" ECG and was told he had evidence of a "heart attack." Note prominent Q waves in leads III and aVF that could easily be misinterpreted

as an inferior MI (due to delta waves distorting the QRS complexes in the inferior leads).

- Pathologic Q waves may be seen in patients with non-ischemic cardiomyopathy, either idiopathic or secondary (e.g., sarcoid, amyloid, tumor, scleroderma), caused by infiltration and/or replacement of the myocardium. An abnormal Q wave in only one lead, however, should be interpreted with caution.
- Pathologic Q waves, ST segment elevation, negative T waves, and QT prolongation may be seen in the absence of fixed CAD in patients with cocaine-induced MI and *stress (Takotsubo) cardiomyopathy* (due to coronary vasospasm or neurogenic myocardial stunning).
- Patients with hypertrophic cardiomyopathy also frequently have abnormal Q waves (due to left to right depolarization of the hypertrophied septum) in the inferior and lateral leads that mimic MI along with LV hypertrophy.
- Giant negative (inverted) T waves in the precordial leads provide clues to the presence of a variant form of hypertrophic cardiomyopathy localized principally to the apex (known as *Yamaguchi syndrome*). *The ECG is a very useful tool in screening for hypertrophic obstructive cardiomyopathy since a normal tracing almost rules out this diagnosis.*
- Giant T wave inversions, known as *cerebral T waves*, and QT prolongation, along with an increase in U wave amplitude and bradycardia, may also be

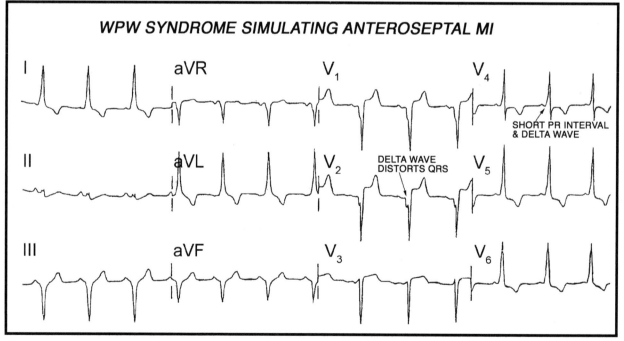

Fig. 3-20.

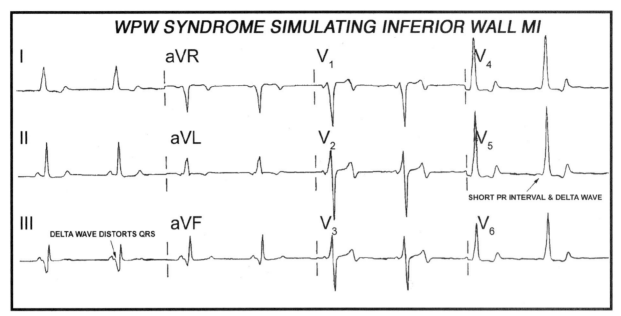

WPW SYNDROME SIMULATING INFERIOR WALL MI

I   aVR   V₁   V₄

II   aVL   V₂   V₅

SHORT PR INTERVAL & DELTA WAVE

III   DELTA WAVE DISTORTS QRS   aVF   V₃   V₆

Fig. 3-21.

seen with central nervous system (CNS) disease, most notably subarachnoid and intracerebral hemorrhages, presumably as a result of autonomic imbalance (**Figure 3-22**).

Figure 3-22. T wave inversions may be seen in a variety of clinical conditions. Note the deep, symmetrically inverted T wave in acute myocardial ischemia (**left**); deep, wide T wave inversion (so-called cerebral T wave) along with prolonged QT interval in central nervous system (CNS) disease (**middle**); and giant negative (inverted) T wave with prominent LV voltage in apical hypertrophic cardiomyopathy (**right**).

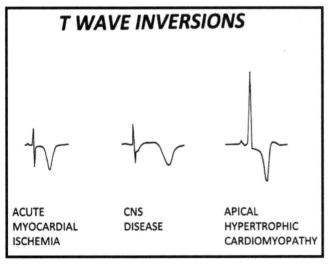

T WAVE INVERSIONS

ACUTE
MYOCARDIAL
ISCHEMIA

CNS
DISEASE

APICAL
HYPERTROPHIC
CARDIOMYOPATHY

Fig. 3-22.

* * *

Pearls:

- All patients presenting with chest pain concerning for acute myocardial ischemia should have an ECG performed and interpreted promptly. If the initial ECG is normal and the patient continues to have symptoms suggestive of ischemia, the ECG should be repeated.

- ST segment changes that accompany ischemic syndromes are due to electrical currents between ischemic and nonischemic regions of the myocardium. The direction of the electrical currents (vector of ST segment displacement) is oriented toward the injured area.

- The magnitude of ST segment deviation correlates with the extent and severity of ischemia. Unlike ST segment elevation, however, ST segment depression does not localize the ischemic territory involved.

- Subendocardial ischemia, as seen in classic angina caused by fixed coronary obstruction, or non-ST segment elevation MI typically shows ST segment depression and symmetric T wave inversion.

- More severe, or transmural, ischemia tends to produce elevation of the ST segment (current of injury pattern) in the ECG leads overlying the affected area, with reciprocal ST segment depression in the opposite leads.

- Prinzmetal's (variant) angina, caused by coronary vasospasm, produces transient ST segment elevation without Q waves.

- In ST segment elevation MI, early "hyperacute" T wave peaking may precede ST segment elevation, which usually develops within minutes, and is followed within hours to days by symmetric T wave inversion, and usually pathologic Q wave formation (a sign of necrosis)
- The specific ECG leads with ST segment elevation can help localize the infarct to the anterior (leads V1-V4), lateral (leads I, aVL, V5 and V6), or inferior (leads II, III, and aVF) portions of the myocardium. In general, the more elevated the ST segments and the more ST segments that are elevated, the more extensive is the infarction.
- Inferior wall MIs can result from occlusion of the right coronary artery, or, less commonly, the left circumflex coronary artery. The presence of ST segment elevation in lead III greater than that in lead II predicts a right coronary artery occlusion. ST segment elevation in at least one lateral lead (I, aVL, V5 or V6) strongly suggests a left circumflex lesion.
- Inferior ST segment elevation should prompt consideration of an associated right ventricular infarction, which may be detected by ST segment elevation in lead V1 or the right sided chest leads (e.g., V4R). When present, it is predictive of a proximal right coronary artery occlusion.
- ST segment depression accompanied by tall R waves in the anterior precordial leads (V1-V3) may reflect reciprocal (mirror image) ECG changes of a posterior wall MI.
- Although patients presenting with an acute MI and new LBBB benefit from rapid reperfusion therapy, LBBB by itself in a patient with chest pain is no longer considered a STEMI equivalent since only a small percentage of these patients are actually having an acute MI. Specific ECG criteria for acute MI in the setting of LBBB (or ventricular paced rhythm) include concordant ST segment elevation (in the same direction as the QRS complex) and excessively discordant ST segment elevation (in the opposite direction of the QRS complex).
- ST segment elevation in lead aVR, particularly in combination with ST segment elevation in V1 and diffuse ST segment depression in multiple other leads, is highly suggestive of ischemia due to occlusion of the left main or proximal left anterior descending coronary artery.
- Patients presenting with chest pain and upsloping ST segment depression accompanied by tall, upright (hyperacute) T waves (de Winter's sign), should receive early attempts at reperfusion since the underlying cause may be an acute coronary occlusion.
- Patients presenting with chest pain accompanied by deep T wave inversion in precordial leads V1-V4 (Wellen's pattern), should receive early interventional management since this ECG pattern is associated with high grade stenosis of the proximal LAD coronary artery.
- Once jeopardized myocardium is reperfused (by PCI or thrombolysis), the ST segment elevation may resolve. T waves usually remain inverted, and Q waves may, or may not, regress.
- In the absence of reperfusion, the ST segment gradually returns to baseline in several hours to days, and T wave inversion may eventually become upright.
- When the ST segment is elevated, the infarction is generally considered acute or recent.
- Persistent ST segment elevation, lasting several weeks or more, may represent ventricular aneurysm formation.
- If a pathologic Q wave is present, but there is no ST segment elevation on the ECG, the infarction is probably old or of indeterminate age.
- It is important not to overinterpret the ECG. The range of normal is broad, and the clinical presentation should dictate the importance of a particular ECG finding.

* * *

4

Cardiac Chamber Enlargement And Hypertrophy

Cardiac chamber enlargement or hypertrophy may involve the atria, the ventricles, or both. It implies either dilatation or thickening of the chamber walls. Although imaging techniques, e.g., echocardiography, are considered more sensitive and specific, the 12-lead ECG still remains a simple screening tool for identifying enlargement or hypertrophy of the cardiac chambers.

Left Atrial and Right Atrial Enlargement

Atrial chamber enlargement is caused by clinical conditions that increase volume and/or pressure overload of the atrium. Atrial enlargement can be diagnosed on the ECG by careful analysis of the P wave. As previously mentioned in **Chapter 2**, an increase in the P wave amplitude to > 2.5 mm in lead II indicates RA enlargement, whereas a broad and notched (*double hump*) P wave in lead II and a wide and deep (> 1mm) biphasic P wave in lead V1 indicate LA enlargement (**Figure 2-4**). The primary cause of RA enlargement (*P pulmonale*) is pulmonary hypertension, as seen in chronic pulmonary disease. LA enlargement (*P mitrale*) is associated with mitral valve disease and conditions that cause LV hypertrophy (see below).

Nowadays, the more general term *atrial abnormality* is commonly used instead of atrial enlargement, since both structural and electrical abnormalities (e.g., intra-atrial conduction delay) can influence the size and shape of the P wave.

Perhaps the least reliable of anatomic diagnoses based on ECG criteria is that of ventricular hypertrophy or enlargement. Very significant degrees of anatomic RV hypertrophy can exist with little or no detectable change in the ECG. In addition, considerable LV hypertrophy can occur with only slight enhancement of the normal LV dominance. Nevertheless, the ECG may offer supporting evidence of LV or RV hypertrophy though it is a relatively insensitive method of detecting it.

Left Ventricular Hypertrophy

Left ventricular hypertrophy is caused by clinical conditions that increase pressure and/or volume overload of the left ventricle. It can be diagnosed by careful analysis of the height (voltage) of the QRS complex.

- For LV hypertrophy, increased voltage amplitude, particularly in the precordial leads, is the most commonly used of all the ECG criteria. According to the *Sokolow-Lyon criteria*, if the sum of the depth of the S wave in lead V1 and the height of the R wave in leads V5 or V6 is greater than 35 mm, then there is evidence of LV hypertrophy. An increase in the QRS voltage height in limb lead aVL >11 mm also indicates LV hypertrophy. Of equal value is evidence of ST-T abnormalities (*LV strain pattern*, i.e., ST segment depression and T wave inversion in the left precordial leads V4-V6) reflecting secondary repolarization changes, in the absence of ischemia or digitalis.

- Voltage criteria for LV hypertrophy, along with ST-T wave changes (*LV strain pattern*) may also provide clues to target organ damage from longstanding hypertension, as well as dilated and/or hypertrophic cardiomyopathy (**Figure 4-1**).

Figure 4-1. 12-lead ECG tracing in a patient with poorly controlled hypertension. Note the increased QRS voltage in the precordial leads with ST depression *(strain pattern)*, broad, notched P wave in lead II and wide, biphasic P wave in lead V1 suggesting left atrial enlargement, and left axis deviation, which are all characteristic features of LV hypertrophy. Although the QS pattern (a single negative wave with no R wave to distinguish whether the deflection is Q or an S wave) in the right precordial leads raises the possibility of anteroseptal MI, it is not unusual for LV hypertrophy by itself to present this way.

- Valvular heart diseases with resultant pressure (stenosis) or volume (regurgitation) overload of the LV can also produce ECG evidence of LV hypertrophy. In valvular aortic stenosis, signs of

LV hypertrophy on the ECG may serve as a clue to a significant degree of outflow tract obstruction. Tall positive T waves may also be seen in LV volume loads due to MR or AR.

The ECG is not sensitive for the detection of small degrees of LV hypertrophy. The diagnosis is best made by echocardiography. Evidence of LV hypertrophy (particularly when associated with ST segment depression) and chamber enlargement on the ECG, however, usually signify an advanced stage of disease (i.e., chronic conditions such as hypertension and severe AS that impose prolonged pressure loads on the heart), with a poorer prognosis. Note that effective treatment of systemic arterial hypertension reduces ECG evidence of LV hypertrophy and decreases the associated risk of cardiovascular mortality.

Although chamber hypertrophy is suggested by specific ECG findings, dilatation (an increase in the internal diameter of the cardiac chamber) cannot be differentiated from actual thickening using the ECG alone. Echocardiography is a much more sensitive diagnostic tool.

Right Ventricular Hypertrophy

Right ventricular hypertrophy is much less common than LV hypertrophy and is usually severe before it causes significant ECG changes. Right ventricular hypertrophy is caused by clinical conditions that increase pressure

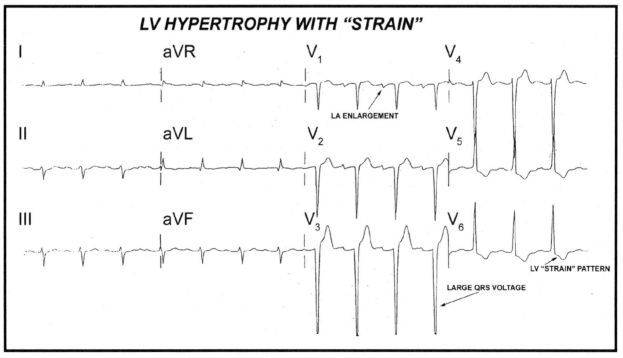

Fig. 4-1.

and/or volume overload of the right ventricle. ECG clues to right ventricular hypertrophy are reflected by changes in the height (voltage) of the QRS complex, as well as a shift in the QRS axis.

- For RV hypertrophy, a combination of right axis deviation with a tall R wave (> 7 mm) and a R/S wave ratio in V1 > 1 and deep S waves in V6 are valuable clues.
- RV hypertrophy can result from a number of conditions that cause pressure and/or volume overload of the RV. These conditions include congenital heart disease: pulmonic valve stenosis, ostium secundum ASD (associated with incomplete or complete RBBB patterns), rheumatic MS, pulmonary hypertension, and lung disease (**Figure 4-2**).

Figure 4-2. 12-lead ECG tracing from a woman with severe pulmonary hypertension. Note the large prominent R wave in lead V1 along with persistent precordial S waves and extreme right axis deviation seen with RV hypertrophy. Tall, peaked P waves in lead II, indicative of RA enlargement (*P pulmonale*) is also present.

- ECG findings of acute RV overload, e.g., right axis deviation, *S1Q3T3 pattern* (deep S wave in lead I, Q wave in lead III and T wave inversion in lead III) in patients with *pulmonary embolism* provide clues to obstruction of >50% of the pulmonary arterial bed and significant pulmonary hypertension (**Figure 4-3**).

Figure 4-3. ECG findings in acute pulmonary embolism. Pulmonary embolism causes acute strain on the right heart and right axis deviation. Note the deep S wave in lead I, along with a Q wave in lead III and T wave inversion in lead III. Although the S1Q3T3 pattern is a classic sign, it only occurs in about 15% of cases. Sinus tachycardia is the most common ECG finding of a pulmonary embolism.

* * *

Pearls:

- RA enlargement produces tall, peaked P waves in lead II. It is referred to as P pulmonale since it may be caused by pulmonary hypertension and severe pulmonary disease.

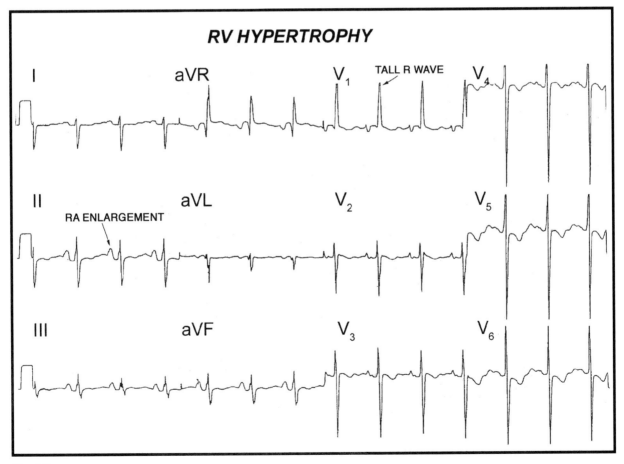

Fig. 4-2.

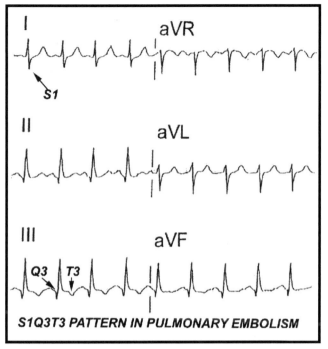

S1Q3T3 PATTERN IN PULMONARY EMBOLISM

Fig. 4-3.

- LA enlargement produces wide, bifid P waves in leads II and VI. It is referred to as P mitrale because it is classically seen in mitral valve disease.
- In LV hypertrophy, leads that "look at" the LV (e.g. V5 and V6) show taller than normal R waves, and leads that "look away" from the LV (e.g., V1) show deeper than normal S waves.
- A simple rule for LV hypertrophy: Add the depth of the S wave in lead V1 and the height of the R wave in lead V5 or V6. If the sum is greater than 35mm, voltage criteria for LV hypertrophy is present.
- In RV hypertrophy, leads that "look at" the RV (e.g., V1) show a tall R wave and leads that "look away" from the RV (e.g., V5 or V6) show a deep S wave.
- A simple rule for RV hypertrophy: A tall R wave in lead V1 + right axis deviation = RV hypertrophy.
- Although the S1Q3T3 pattern is a classic ECG sign of pulmonary embolism, it is seen in only a minority of cases. Sinus tachycardia is the most common ECG finding of a pulmonary embolism.

* * *

5

Arrhythmias and Conduction Disturbances

Disorders of heart rate and rhythm result from alterations of impulse formation and/or conduction. The presentation of arrhythmias may range from common benign palpitations to severe life-threatening rhythm disturbances that impair normal cardiac output.

A patient's awareness of palpitations (and of regular or irregular cardiac rhythm) varies significantly. Some patients perceive slight variations in their heart rhythm with great accuracy, whereas others are oblivious even to sustained episodes of VT. Still others complain of palpitations when they actually are in normal sinus rhythm. What is palpitation to one patient, therefore, may not be to another. Some patients may be able to use their hand to "tap out" what they feel (or recognize the beat "tapped out" by the clinician's hand) and thus identify their arrhythmia.

Figure 5-1. Using your hand to tap out the heartbeat is a useful technique to help simulate and diagnose various arrhythmias. Note the clinician's hand is moving up and down rapidly to indicate a tachycardia. **A.** Premature ventricular contraction (3rd beat); **B.** Supraventricular tachycardia; **C.** Atrial flutter; **D.** Atrial fibrillation; **E.** Ventricular tachycardia.

The sensitivity and specificity of ECG changes for cardiac rhythm and conduction abnormalities are relatively high and provide clues to the origins of palpitations, dizziness, or syncope. The causes may include:

- Atrial and/or ventricular extrasystoles
- Significant tachy- or bradyarrhythmias
- Mobitz type I (Wenckebach) second-degree AV block (gradually increasing PR interval with eventual dropped beat)
- Mobitz type II second-degree AV block (fixed PR interval with abrupt dropped beat)
- Complete heart block (changing PR intervals with complete lack of communication between P and QRS)
- Right or left bundle branch block
- Wolff-Parkinson-White (WPW) syndrome with its associated risk of atrioventricular reentry tachycardia
- Long QT interval (e.g., resulting from antiarrhythmic agents, hypokalemia, hypomagnesemia, tricyclic antidepressants) with its attendant risk of polymorphic ventricular tachycardia (*torsades de pointes*)

Figure 5-2. Palpitations described as a "flip-flop sensation" or a "skip" (something "turned over in my chest") suggest early extra heartbeats, either PACs (**top**) or PVCs (**bottom**). This usually represents awareness of the more forceful beat that occurs after the pause rather than the premature beat itself. The post-extrasystolic pause may be perceived as an actual cessation of heartbeat ("my heart stopped"). Premature ectopic beats

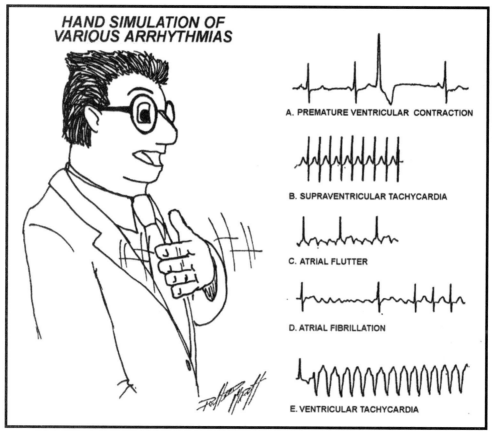

Fig. 5-1.

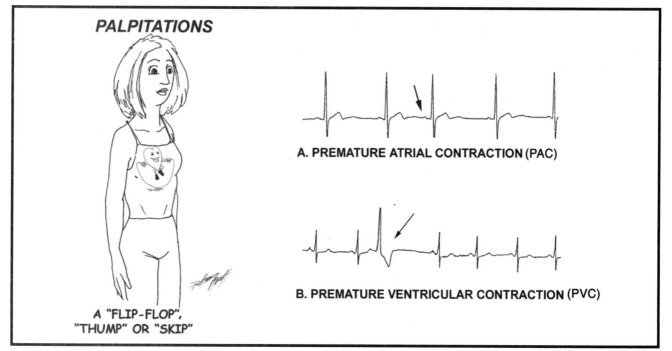

Fig. 5-2.

occur commonly, both in the presence and absence of heart disease.

Mechanisms of Arrhythmias

In general, it is first helpful to note whether there is a bradycardia (slow heart rhythm) or a tachycardia (fast heart rhythm). Bradycardias may originate from an overactive parasympathetic nervous system (e.g., in a trained athlete), a sick sinus node, or a defect in the conduction of impulses from the atria to the ventricles. Sinus bradycardia is common in many normal individuals during sleep.

Tachycardias may originate from an overactive sympathetic nervous system, hyperactivity of the SA node in response to either a physiologic state (e.g., exercise, anxiety) or a pathophysiologic condition (e.g., fever, pulmonary embolus), ectopic atrial pacemakers, hyperactive cardiac conduction system (e.g., irritable focus in the bundle of His), or irritable focus in the ventricular myocardium. Sympathetic stimulation, hyperthyroidism, digitalis toxicity, caffeine, ethanol, amphetamines, cocaine, and, to some degree, low O_2 can cause irritability of the atrial and conduction system foci. Hypoxia and low potassium are more likely causes of ventricular irritability, but adrenergic stimulants can also irritate ventricular foci.

Cardiac arrhythmias may result from 3 mechanisms:

1. *Abnormal automaticity* (electrical impulses arise spontaneously)
2. *Triggered activity* (impulses caused by afterdepolarizations [i.e., oscillations of the membrane potential] of a preceding impulse), and most commonly
3. *Reentry* (impulses travel in a self-perpetuating, circular loop [so-called circus movement] to re-excite the same region)

It is helpful to note whether the arrhythmia involves a normal narrow QRS complex or a wide QRS complex. Narrow complex arrhythmias imply that the problem is not in the ventricular myocardium, since abnormal discharges there result in bizarre wide QRS complexes. Wide QRS complexes imply that the atria are not the sole origin of the arrhythmia; there is some other deficit, whether in the conduction system, involving a blockage somewhere in the conduction system (e.g., RBBB or LBBB) or an aberrant reentry circuit, or an abnormal focus in the ventricular myocardium.

Figure 5-3. An arrhythmia that originates above the ventricles in the atria or atrioventricular (AV) node is called a *supraventricular arrhythmia*. This figure shows the mechanisms of various supraventricular tachyarrhythmias and their corresponding ECG features. **Left Top.** In *AV nodal reentry tachycardia*, the QRS complexes are regular, and the P waves are usually buried in or distort the terminal portion of the QRS. Reentry occurs using dual pathways in the AV node. **Left Bottom.** In *atrial fibrillation*, the QRS complexes are irregularly irregular, and no organized P waves are seen. Multiple reentry sites (*wavelets*) in the atria fire impulses in an uncoordinated fashion down the AV node. **Right Top.** In *atrial flutter*, the contractions of the atrium are more coordinated, involving macroreentry (a larger reentrant circuit) in the right atrium, and the

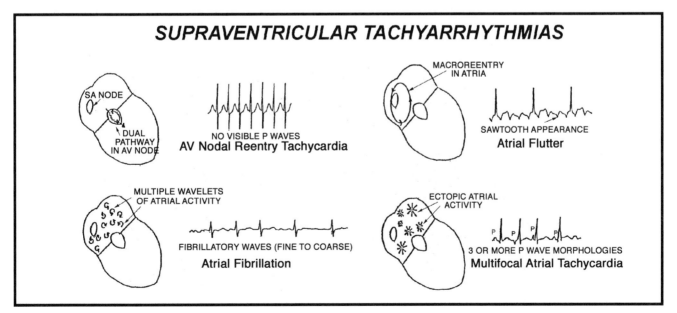

Fig. 5-3.

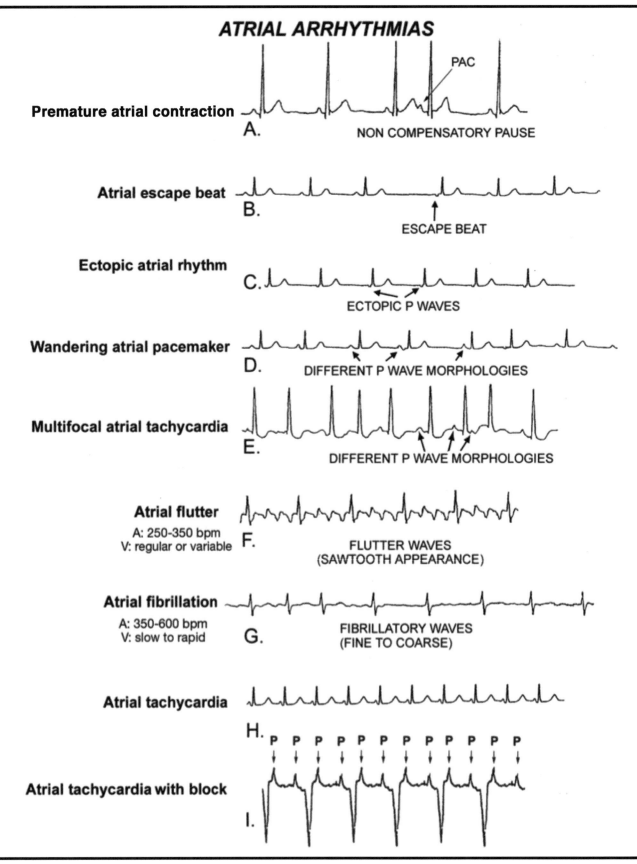

Fig. 5-4.

heart rhythm tends to be regular. The *sawtooth pattern* of flutter waves is best seen in the inferior leads. **Right Bottom**. In *multifocal atrial tachycardia*, 3 or more P waves of differing morphologies are present. There is increased automaticity at multiple sites in the atria, and the rhythm is irregular.

In most cases, logical reasoning should enable you to determine whether the arrhythmia originates in the atria, ventricles or conduction system.

Supraventricular Arrhythmias

Figure 5-4 shows many different kinds of atrial arrhythmias:

A. *Premature atrial contraction (PAC).* Early ectopic beat originates in atria not in sinus node, resulting in a short PR interval, since a number of potential atrial ectopic foci lie around the coronary sinus, the myocardial venous drainage channel, which empties into the right atrium and lies near the AV node. PACs typically present as a narrow complex QRS preceded by a premature P wave. Sometimes there may be a slight widening of the QRS (PAC with aberrancy), if one of the bundle branches (usually the right) is not yet repolarized when the atrial impulse gets through (so-called *Ashman phenomenon*). Although aberration may be seen during PACs, it can also occur after a long-short R-R interval in atrial fibrillation. PACs may be single, occur in pairs (*couplets*), or three in a row (*triplets*). They may arise from one ectopic focus (*unifocal*) or from two or more ectopic foci (*multifocal*). PACs may also occur in a rhythmic sequence alternating with a normal beat. This is called *bigeminy* if every other beat is premature, *trigeminy* if every third beat is premature, and so forth. PACs usually reset the sinus mechanism and are not followed by a compensatory pause (i.e., the P wave following the PAC occurs at less than twice the normal P-P interval). If the ectopic atrial focus fires very soon after the previous beat, the impulse may encounter an AV node that is still refractory to excitation, resulting in a blocked PAC that does not conduct to the ventricles (the ectopic P wave will not be followed by a QRS complex). Keep in mind that the most common unexpected pause is due to a non-conducted PAC.

B. *Atrial escape beat.* Occurs when the sinus node is firing so slowly that an ectopic focus in the atrium acts to fill in a beat.

C. *Ectopic atrial rhythm.* The rhythm originates from an ectopic focus in the atrium, resulting in a short PR interval, since the ectopic focus is closer to the AV node. (Note that the P wave may not be upright in lead II in ectopic atrial rhythm.)

D. *Wandering atrial pacemaker.* The atria are activated by multiple foci, resulting in changes in P waves on the ECG. The rate is typically less than 100 beats/min. When it exceeds that, it is called *multifocal atrial tachycardia (MAT)*, which is not uncommon in chronic obstructive pulmonary disease (COPD).

E. *Multifocal atrial tachycardia.* Note more than 3 different P wave morphologies and varying PR intervals due to each complex originating from different foci in the atria. A flat isoelectric baseline between the P waves distinguishes MAT from atrial fibrillation.

F. *Atrial flutter* with 4:1 AV conduction. Note the *sawtooth pattern* of flutter waves due to continuous circus movement of the electrical wave form (macro-reentry) within the atrium. Typical atrial firing rates in atrial flutter are 250-350/min with varying ventricular responses.

G. *Atrial fibrillation.* An irregularly irregular rhythm with no organized atrial activity and no effective mechanical atrial contraction. Note irregular fibrillatory waves arising in atria. Typical atrial firing rates in atrial fibrillation are 350-600/min with varying ventricular responses. When atrial fibrillation is detected on the ECG, you should consider the possibility of mitral valve disease, hyperthyroidism, alcohol consumption, pericardial disease, or atrial septal defect. Other conditions that increase atrial pressure and size, including CHF, hypertension, CAD, cardiomyopathy, and pulmonary disease may also cause atrial fibrillation.

H. *Atrial tachycardia (AT).* A rapid, regular atrial rhythm at a rate of 150-250/min, generally originating from an ectopic atrial focus or reentry within the atria.

I. *Atrial tachycardia (AT) with block.* The atrial firing rate may be so fast that not every impulse can get through to the ventricles (commonly seen in the presence of digitalis toxicity). In this case, there are 2 P waves for every QRS complex.

AV Junctional Arrhythmias

Figure 5-5. Arrhythmias may also originate from junctional (AV nodal) irritability:

A. *Junctional escape beat.* An escape beat that originates in the AV node secondary to depression of the higher sinus pacemaker. The QRS may be slightly prolonged in cases where a bundle branch is not

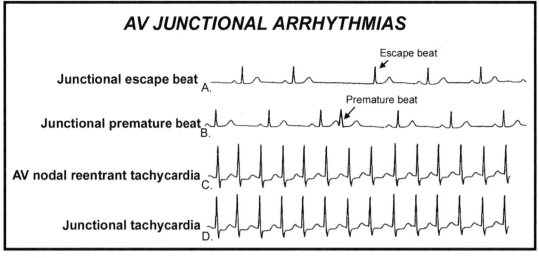

AV JUNCTIONAL ARRHYTHMIAS

Junctional escape beat A.

Escape beat

Junctional premature beat B.

Premature beat

AV nodal reentrant tachycardia C.

Junctional tachycardia D.

Fig. 5-5.

completely repolarized at the time the premature impulse comes through the bundle of His.

B. *Junctional premature beat.* A premature, ectopic supraventricular impulse that originates from the area in and around the AV node. A visible P wave may or may not be present. If visible, the P wave commonly occurs just before (short PR interval) or just after the QRS complex and is inverted in leads II, III, and aVF, indicating an origin low down in the atria, at the AV junction.

C. *AV nodal reentrant tachycardia* (at rates of 150-250/min) looks similar on ECG to that of paroxysmal junctional tachycardia. It is driven by a reentry circus loop within the AV node. P waves may not be seen, or they may be inverted (before or after the QRS) due to retrograde transmission to the atria.

D. *Junctional tachycardia* occurs when a tachycardia is driven by an irritable focus within the AV node. P waves may not be seen, or they may be inverted (before or after the QRS) due to retrograde transmission to the atria.

Figure 5-6. Arrhythmias seen in digitalis toxicity are thought to be due to triggered activity caused by delayed afterdepolarizations plus suppression of sinus and AV nodal pacemaker function. These include paroxysmal atrial tachycardia with AV block, bidirectional VT (QRS complexes from two different ectopic foci alternate in morphology, and "regularization" of atrial fibrillation (regular R-R intervals) due to a junctional rhythm and AV dissociation. Concave or "scooped" ST segment depression is seen with therapeutic levels of digitalis (so-called *digitalis effect*) and is not indicative of digitalis toxicity.

Figure 5-7. Schematic illustration of typical mechanism of supraventricular tachycardia due to AV nodal reentry using dual pathways in the AV node. α fibers = slow pathway, β fibers = fast pathway that was previously blocked. Supraventricular tachycardia is a rapid and regular heart rhythm that begins and ends abruptly. Heart rate may be 150-250 beats/min.

Paroxysmal SVT occurs in individuals of all ages, and is often seen in otherwise healthy young adult females without underlying structural heart disease. *AV nodal reentrant tachycardia (AVNRT)* is the most common type of paroxysmal SVT, occurring in 50–60% of cases. The reentry circuit is located within the AV node with impulses traveling down the slow (α) pathway and then retrograde up the fast (β) pathway of the AV node (**Figure 5-7**). The atria and ventricles are depolarized simultaneously, and the P waves are hidden in the QRS complexes on the ECG. The episode usually begins and ends abruptly and may last seconds to several hours or longer. The QRS complexes are typically narrow.

AV reciprocating tachycardia (AVRT), which includes WPW, is the second most common form of paroxysmal SVT (30–40% of cases) and most commonly utilizes the normal AV pathway and an accessory bypass tract for antegrade and/or retrograde conduction (preexcitation [WPW] syndrome). About one half of patients with the WPW pattern on a routine ECG have periodic tachyarrhythmias, whereas the other half demonstrate no rhythm disturbances. In some patients with this syndrome, the characteristic ECG features (short PR interval, delta wave) occur intermittently, or not at all. In these patients, the accessory pathway functions only in the retrograde direction (i.e., *concealed*), so that the QRS complexes are electrocardiographically normal.

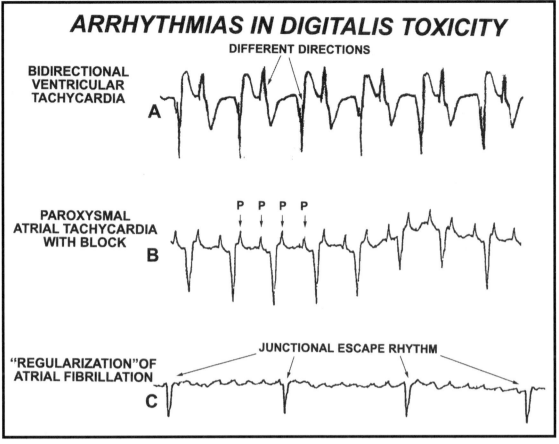

Fig. 5-6.

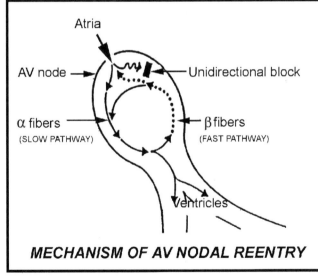

MECHANISM OF AV NODAL REENTRY

Fig. 5-7.

Frequently, the first episode of AVNRT occurs before the age of 30 although it may start after the patient has reached 60 years of age. AVNRT is characterized by the sudden onset and offset of a regular tachycardia at rates of 150 to 250 beats per minute. Many attacks

of paroxysmal SVT resolve spontaneously. If not, vagal maneuvers (e.g., Valsalva maneuver, carotid sinus massage, breath holding, immersing the face in ice water) may terminate the attack. *Response to vagal maneuvers may be diagnostic since paroxysmal SVT is, with rare exception, the only tachycardia that can be broken and stay normal during these maneuvers.*

Vagal Maneuvers

Vagal maneuvers work by slowing the rate at which the sinus node fires and, more importantly, by blocking conduction through the AV node (thereby breaking the reentry circuit).

Carotid sinus massage is a simple and useful vagotonic maneuver to diagnose and/or treat various tachyarrhythmias. This maneuver stimulates the baroreceptor reflex, which elicits an increase in vagal tone. Before commencing with this maneuver, however, palpate and listen for carotid bruits to exclude carotid artery stenosis. This finding, along with a history of TIAs, are contraindications for carotid sinus massage. Massage one side of the neck at a time, *never both carotids at the same time!* Your patient's head should be turned to the left and the right carotid artery palpated high in the neck, at the angle of the jaw (where the carotid sinus is located). While listening with your stethoscope over the patient's chest (and/or recording the procedure with constant ECG monitoring), press this area firmly for 3–5 seconds at a time with either your index and middle fingers, or with your thumb. Stop the pressure immediately if a response is obtained. Do not use prolonged carotid sinus stimulation, since serious consequences (e.g., prolonged asystole) may occur. Repeat as necessary. It is important to apply sufficient pressure, which will usually cause some discomfort to the patient (of which the patient should be warned).

When carotid sinus massage is not effective, it may mean that the exact spot at the angle of the jaw has not been located, and that you need to reposition your fingers or move to the left side. Keep in mind that slowing (e.g., sinus tachycardia, atrial flutter/fibrillation) or conversion (e.g., supraventricular tachycardia) of the ventricular rate with carotid sinus pressure rules out the most serious arrhythmia, VT, which generally will not respond.

Figure 5-8. Left. Technique of carotid sinus massage. The patient's head is tilted backward and to the left. The practitioner's hand applies pressure with the thumb to the carotid artery pulsation just under the angle of the right jaw. The procedure is monitored by listening with the stethoscope and/or by continuous ECG recording.

Right. Effect of carotid sinus pressure on various tachycardias. (Courtesy of Dr. W. Proctor Harvey). **Note** the effect of carotid sinus massage on each type of tachycardia:

- There is a gradual slowing and gradual return to former rate with *sinus tachycardia*.

- *AV nodal reentrant tachycardia (AVNRT)* is abruptly stopped, followed by normal sinus rhythm.
- *Atrial fibrillation*. Rate is originally irregular and rapid; there is immediate slowing with irregular return to former rhythm.
- There is prompt slowing with irregular "jerky" return to original 2:1 *atrial flutter*. The atria remain undisturbed.
- With *paroxysmal atrial tachycardia (PAT) with block* (not every P wave gets through in this tachyarrhythmia), carotid pressure produces slowing. Note atrial waves easily identified.
- There is no effect whatsoever on *ventricular tachycardia*.

Figure 5-9. Wolff-Parkinson-White (WPW) syndrome. Conduction occurs through an accessory pathway between the atria and ventricles (so-called *Bundle of Kent*) as well as the normal pathway via the AV node. The accessory pathway starts stimulating the ventricle early (*preexcitation*), and the combination of accessory and normal pathways results in a widened QRS and a shortened PR interval. Note the short PR interval, due to rapid conduction through the accessory pathway, slurred upstroke of the QRS complex (*delta wave*), and prolonged QRS secondary to slow ventricular activation. There may also be an inverted T wave. WPW may also present as a tachycardia, with a reentry circuit loop. Whether the reentry tachycardia is associated with a narrow (normal) or a wide QRS complex is determined by whether antegrade conduction is through the AV node (normal QRS width) – "orthodromic" AV reentry tachycardia, or through the accessory pathway (widened QRS complex due to the aberrant route though the ventricles) – "antidromic" AV reentry tachycardia. The latter arrhythmia is difficult to distinguish from VT.

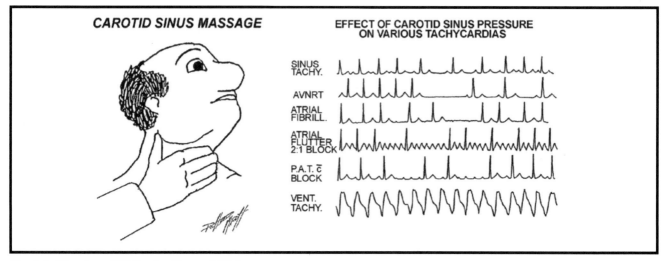

Fig. 5-8. (Courtesy of W. Proctor Harvey, M.D.)

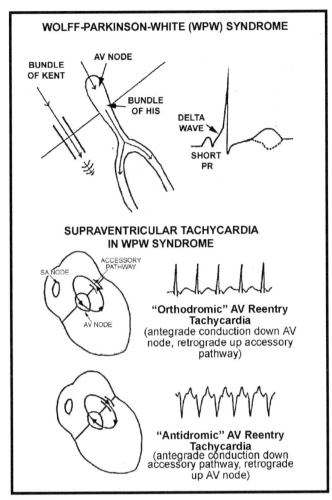

WOLFF-PARKINSON-WHITE (WPW) SYNDROME

BUNDLE OF KENT

AV NODE

BUNDLE OF HIS

DELTA WAVE

SHORT PR

SUPRAVENTRICULAR TACHYCARDIA IN WPW SYNDROME

SA NODE

ACCESSORY PATHWAY

AV NODE

"Orthodromic" AV Reentry Tachycardia
(antegrade conduction down AV node, retrograde up accessory pathway)

"Antidromic" AV Reentry Tachycardia
(antegrade conduction down accessory pathway, retrograde up AV node)

Fig. 5-9.

Figure 5-10. ECG tracing of atrial fibrillation conducted down an accessory pathway in a patient with *preexcitation (WPW) syndrome*. The presence of a ventricular rate >200 beats/min in the setting of atrial fibrillation provides a clue to WPW (and a bypass tract that circumvents the AV node) since it is unlikely that the AV node will conduct more than 200 impulses per minute. This arrhythmia can degenerate into ventricular fibrillation if AV nodal blocking agents (e.g., digoxin, verapamil, beta blockers) are administered, which block the AV node and allow more conduction through the bypass tract.

Figure 5-11. Top. Schematic representation of rapid atrial fibrillation in preexcitation (WPW) syndrome. Note very rapid ventricular rate and bizarre-looking wide QRS complexes (so-called *wacky-cardia*) that can mimic polymorphic ventricular tachycardia (*torsades de pointes*) (**bottom**) as seen in patients with long QT syndrome. Keep in mind the possibility of preexcited atrial fibrillation in any young patient who presents to the Emergency Department with a rapid, irregular wide complex tachycardia. Rapid atrial fibrillation in such a patient can result in ventricular fibrillation if AV nodal blocking agents (e.g., digitalis, beta blocker, verapamil) are administered. (These AV nodal blocking agents increase the refractory period in the AV node and paradoxically allow even more atrial impulses to get through the accessory pathway to the ventricle.) These patients require careful evaluation and electrophysiologic study.

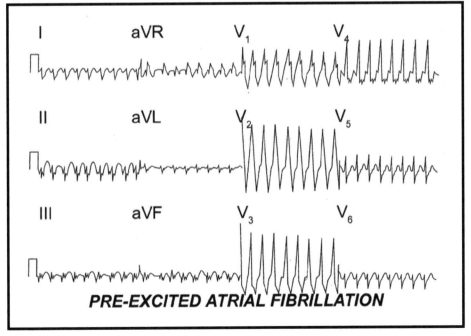

I aVR V₁ V₄

II aVL V₂ V₅

III aVF V₃ V₆

PRE-EXCITED ATRIAL FIBRILLATION

Fig. 5-10.

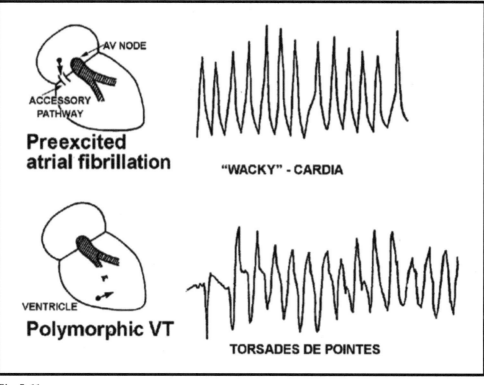

Fig. 5-11.

Figure 5-12. 12-lead ECG in a patient with a history of palpitations and WPW. Note the short PR interval (e.g., lead II) and delta wave.

WPW patterns on the ECG are divided into two types: Type A (predominantly positive delta wave and QRS complex in the chest leads) and Type B (predominantly negative delta wave and QRS complex in leads V1 and V2).

The accessory pathway bypasses the AV node and rapidly conducts the impulse directly from the atria to the ventricles, producing early depolarization, or *preexcitation* (a kind of electrical "short circuit" manifested by the classic delta wave). The position of the accessory pathway can be accurately localized only with electrophysiologic studies. In general, however, a dominant S wave in leads V1-V3 indicates a right-sided pathway, whereas a dominant R wave in leads V1-V3 indicates a left-sided pathway. Although the presence of an accessory pathway may be detected on an ECG, the accessory pathway may, at times, be hidden from view, i.e., *concealed*, if it conducts only in a retrograde direction. Furthermore, not everyone with WPW will develop tachycardia or require special treatment.

Figure 5-13. Lown-Ganong-Levine (LGL) syndrome. Atrial impulses may bypass the AV node using a fast-conducting accessory pathway (atrio-His fibers called *James fibers*), but rejoin the bundle of His, thereby producing a short PR interval but normal QRS complex (no delta wave). A tachyarrhythmia may result if impulses spread backward along the rapidly conducting accessory pathway to stimulate the atria at a rapid rate. Patients with a short PR interval on the ECG are prone to atrial reentrant tachyarrhythmias.

Ventricular Arrhythmias

Ventricular arrhythmias originate within the His-Purkinje system or ventricles. Intraventricular conduction is abnormal, resulting in a wide QRS complex. Ventricular arrhythmias originating in the left ventricle generally have an RBBB pattern (positive in V1). Those originating in the right ventricle have an LBBB pattern (negative in V1).

Figure 5-14 shows many different kinds of ventricular arrhythmias:

A. *Premature ventricular contraction (PVC).* Early beat is wide with full compensatory pause between normal beats (i.e., the P wave following the PVC occurs at twice the normal P-P interval). PVCs usually do not reset the atrial rate and are frequently followed by a compensatory pause. PVCs may occur individually, in couplets, or in triplets or salvos, i.e., ventricular tachycardia (see below). Occasionally, the PVC is so premature that the

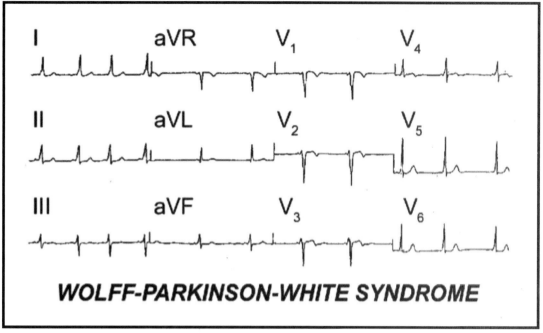

Fig. 5-12.

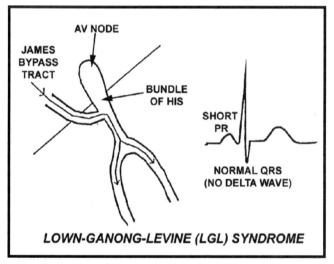

Fig. 5-13.

next sinus impulse finds the ventricle sufficiently recovered to respond. When no compensatory pause occurs, the PVC is termed *interpolated*.

B. *Ventricular escape beat*. Escape beat accommodates for too long a delay in receiving an impulse through the conduction system.

C. *Ventricular bigeminy*. Fixed coupling of independently firing atrial and ventricular complexes. The pattern may also be that of trigeminy (2 normal QRS complexes for every ectopic one) or quadrigeminy (3:1 ratio) with increasing ratio of normal to abnormal QRS complexes.

D. *Ventricular parasystole*. An automatic ventricular focus with entrance block (i.e., the focus is

"protected" and is not depolarized by the natural pacemaker or other outside impulses), creating an independent ectopic ventricular rhythm occurring alongside the native dominant rhythm. In ventricular parasystole, the independent ectopic rhythm is not associated with the underlying sinus rhythm. Ectopic QRS complexes occur at fixed intervals or multiples of a common denominator. The distance between any 2 ectopic beats (the *interectopic interval*) is a multiple of the shortest distance between 2 ectopic beats.

E. *Multifocal PVCs* occur when there is more than one irritable foci. The PVCs are of different shape.

F. *Accelerated idioventricular rhythm*. Idioventricular rhythm is paced by the ventricle at 20-40 firings/min, in the absence of input from the SA node. When the rhythm is greater than 40/min, it is termed an *accelerated idioventricular rhythm* or "slow VT" (see below). Note *fusion beat* (second complex) (signifying a P wave that got through the AV node to generate part of a normal QRS complex that fuses with an abnormal ventricular complex).

G. *Monomorphic ventricular tachycardia (VT)*. VT is a rapid succession of 3 or more beats that originate in the ventricle, either from an ectopic focus or reentry in the ventricle. VT is either nonsustained (lasts <30 seconds) or sustained (lasts ≥30 seconds). Note the rapid succession of wide QRS complexes at rates of 150-250/min. Ventricular flutter (rates of 250-350/min) can look like a very fast ventricular tachycardia and commonly degenerates into ventricular fibrillation. Although

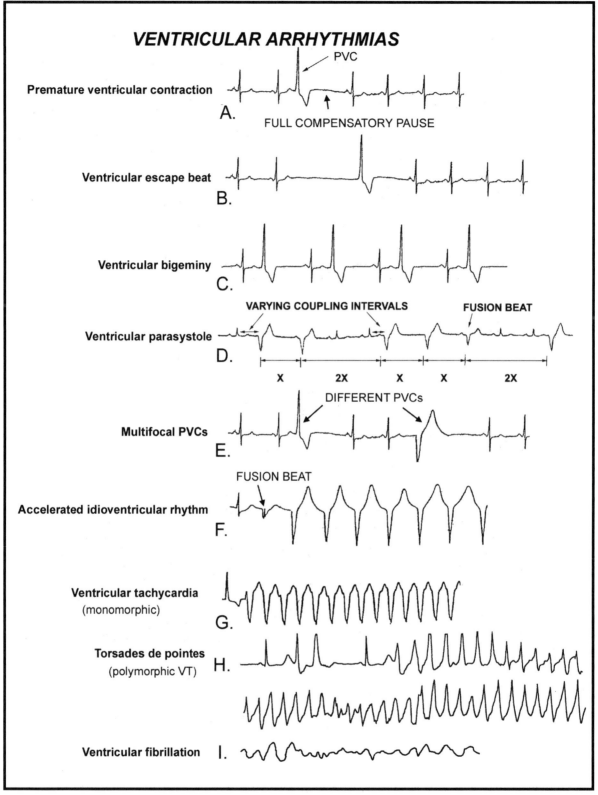

Fig. 5-14.

VT can occur in patients without structural heart disease, common causes include acute myocardial ischemia and infarction, cardiomyopathy, CHF, and digitalis toxicity.

H. *Polymorphic ventricular tachycardia* with long QT interval (*torsades de pointes*). A form of ventricular tachycardia (due to triggered activity caused by early afterdepolarizations) in which the QRS complex morphology varies (PVCs arise from a changing ectopic focus) and twists around the baseline. Note alternating negative and positive deflections. This patient had *long QT syndrome*, which predisposes to this arrhythmia. Note that a premature ventricular complex occurring in the T wave (*R on T phenomenon*) provokes the arrhythmia.

I. *Ventricular fibrillation (VF).* A catastrophic dysrhythmia categorized by total disorganization of electrical activity in the heart, resulting in cardiac arrest. There are no identifiable ECG wave forms, and the baseline is undulating and wavy due to deflections (fibrillatory waves) that vary in amplitude and morphology. Large fibrillatory waves characterize *coarse VF*, and small fibrillatory waves characterize *fine VF*, which can degenerate to a "flat line," called asystole (ventricular standstill).

Figure 5-15. ECG tracing demonstrating ventricular tachycardia. Note capture beat (3rd complex) and fusion beat (4th complex, also known as *Dressler's beat)*, characteristic of this dysrhythmia. A capture beat is a normal QRS complex arising when an atrial impulse succeeds in getting through the AV node to accompany the abnormal PVC-type complexes of a ventricular tachycardia. A fusion beat occurs when the impulse that got through fuses with a PVC-type complex of the ventricular tachycardia to form a hybrid.

Figure 5-16. Top. ECG tracing showing monomorphic ventricular tachycardia in a patient with CAD. All the QRS complexes have the same configuration. Note that the 2nd beat is a fusion beat.

Bottom. ECG tracing (lead V1) demonstrating wide complex tachycardia with dissociation of the P waves from the QRS complexes, which strongly suggests the diagnosis of VT.

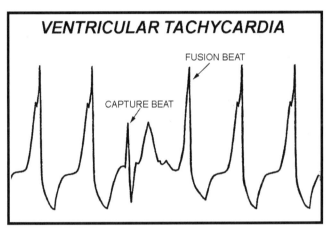

Fig. 5-15.

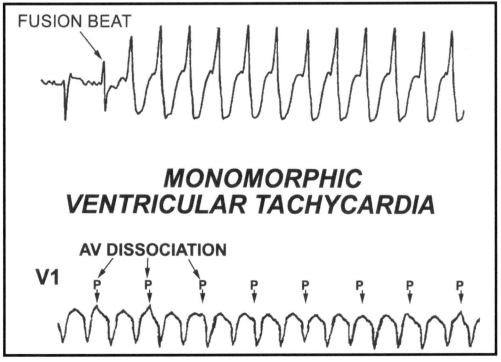

Fig. 5-16.

55

VT can be difficult to distinguish from SVT with aberrancy. Relatively simple ECG criteria (so-called *Brugada criteria*) for differentiating VT from SVT with aberrancy include the following: (1) AV dissociation, (2) QRS morphology inconsistent with a typical RBBB or LBBB, (3) Onset of R-to-nadir of S >100 msec in any precordial lead, and (4) Monophasic QRS concordance (in the same direction) in all precordial leads. The presence of any of these 4 features is diagnostic of VT with a high sensitivity and specificity.

Clues that help differentiate VT from SVT with aberrancy are summarized in **Figure 5-17**.

Electrical Cardioversion and Defibrillation

Tachyarrhythmias (supraventricular or ventricular) that produce chest pain, shortness of breath, decreased level of consciousness, hypotension, shock, CHF, or acute myocardial ischemia may require emergency cardioversion. External cardioversion rapidly establishes normal sinus rhythm. In elective circumstances, cardioversion should always be performed in the synchronized mode (*synchronized to the QRS complex and not on the T wave, which may precipitate VF*).

Figure 5-18. The antero-apical position for cardioversion or defibrillation. Proper electrode position is key.

Figure 5-19. Left parasternal antero-posterior electrode placement for synchronized direct current (DC) cardioversion. This provides optimal current flow

FIGURE 5-17 CLINICAL CLUES TO WIDE COMPLEX TACHYCARDIA	
Supraventricular Tachycardia	**Ventricular Tachycardia**
• Irregularly irregular rhythm • Typical RBBB or LBBB morphology • QRS <0.14 sec (RBBB) or <0.16 sec (LBBB) • History of SVT or WPW syndrome • QRS unchanged or slightly wider than in sinus rhythm • All or none response to carotid sinus massage	• AV dissociation (e.g., independent P waves, capture or fusion beats) • Atypical RBBB or LBBB morphology* • QRS >0.14 sec (RBBB type) or >0.16 sec (LBBB Type) • Positive (or negative) QRS concordance in chest leads • QRS axis −60° to −180° • Presence of heart disease (prior MI, CHF, LV dysfunction)

Note: Assume all wide complex tachycardia is ventricular tachycardia until proven otherwise. The overall appearance of the patient and the hemodynamic stability of the rhythm (presence or absence of hypotension, dizziness, or syncope) do not reliably distinguish ventricular from supraventricular tachycardia. Termination of a wide complex tachycardia by physical maneuvers (e.g., carotid sinus massage, Valsalva) or medication (adenosine) is highly suggestive of SVT.

*In RBBB-type VT, atypical BBB morphology includes a monophasic R wave or an initial R > r' in V1, and a small r and large S wave (r/S ratio < 1) in V6.

In LBBB-type VT, there is an initial r wave > 30 msec in V1, and the onset of QRS to the nadir of S wave (RS interval) > 60-100 msec with a notched or slurred S wave in V1, and a q wave in V6.

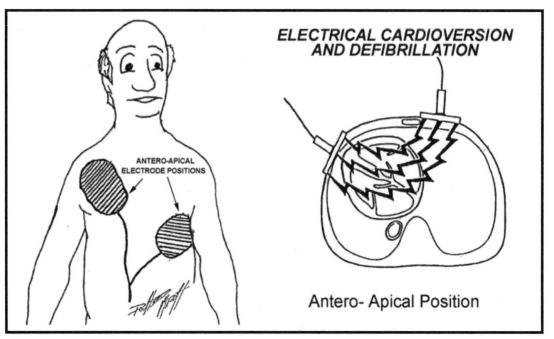

ELECTRICAL CARDIOVERSION AND DEFIBRILLATION

ANTERO-APICAL ELECTRODE POSITIONS

Antero- Apical Position

Fig. 5-18.

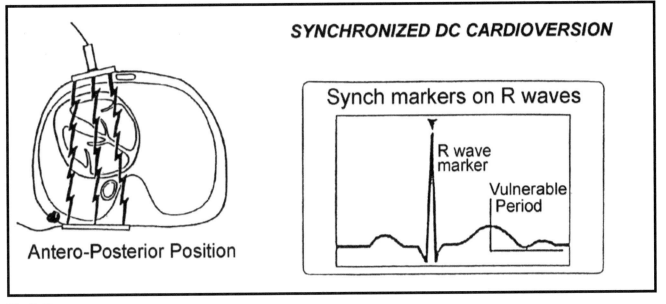

SYNCHRONIZED DC CARDIOVERSION

Antero-Posterior Position

Synch markers on R waves

R wave marker

Vulnerable Period

Fig. 5-19.

through atria and is more effective for cardioversion of atrial fibrillation (courtesy of Dr. Gordon A. Ewy).

Electrical *cardioversion* (shock delivered synchronously with the QRS complex, thus avoiding the vulnerable phase of the cardiac cycle) and *defibrillation* (shock delivered on an emergency basis during cardiac arrest without synchronization to the QRS complex to terminate VF) appear to terminate most effectively those tachycardias presumed to be due to reentry. Reentry tachycardias include atrial flutter and fibrillation, AV nodal reentry, reciprocating tachycardias associated with WPW syndrome, most forms of VT, ventricular flutter and VF. Generally, any tachycardia that produces hypotension, CHF, or angina, and that does not respond quickly and appropriately to medical management should be terminated electrically. When evaluating if a patient is unstable and needs cardioversion, keep in mind the **mnemonic** "CASH": **C**hest pain, **A**ltered mental status, **S**hortness of breath, and **H**ypotension. (You don't get the jewels [joules] if you don't have the cash!) Electrical cardioversion restores normal sinus rhythm in 70% to 95% of patients (depending on the type of tachyarrhythmia).

Bradyarrhythmias and Heart Block

Bradyarrhythmias are common, especially in young, athletic individuals. They are usually due to increased vagal tone and do not require intervention. Abnormalities of conduction can occur between the sinus node and atrium, within the AV node, and in the intraventricular

conduction pathways. Bradyarrhythmias due to these abnormalities may occur with aging and are usually due to idiopathic fibrosis in the conduction tissue (*Lenegre's disease*) or calcification of the cardiac skeleton (*Lev's disease*), CAD, cardiac trauma (postcardiac surgery/ TAVR), tumors, infections (endocarditis, Chagas, Lyme), or other inflammatory or infiltrative disease (e.g., amyloid, sarcoid).

Abnormalities of the cardiac conduction system may result in three general clinical syndromes:

- The *sick sinus syndrome* (which includes marked sinus bradycardia, sinoatrial exit block or arrest, and the so-called *tachy-brady syndrome*)
- *AV nodal-His heart block*
- *Intraventricular (bundle branch) block*

Patients with bradyarrhythmias and conduction abnormalities may be asymptomatic, or present with syncope, near-syncope, lightheadedness, worsening CHF or angina.

Figure 5-20. Sick sinus syndrome. The ECG tracing may show severe *sinus bradycardia* (**top**) or prolonged *sinus pauses* (**middle**) due to *sinus arrest* (a temporary failure of depolarization from the SA node) or *SA exit block* (a temporary failure of the SA nodal impulse to transmit out and into the atria). Sinus arrest and SA exit block result in no depolarization of the atria and absence of the entire P-QRS-T complex. When SA exit block resolves, depolarization of the atria resumes. Since the intrinsic rhythm of the SA node is maintained, the P wave appears in the expected place. The P-P interval surrounding the pause is commonly a multiple of the previous P-P intervals. In contrast, in sinus arrest the SA

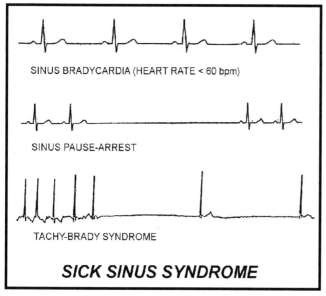

SINUS BRADYCARDIA (HEART RATE < 60 bpm)

SINUS PAUSE-ARREST

TACHY-BRADY SYNDROME

SICK SINUS SYNDROME

Fig. 5-20.

nodal rhythm is reset, and so the reappearance of the P wave is unpredictable. **Bottom.** ECG strip of a patient with *tachy-brady syndrome*. Note the tachycardia component is paroxysmal atrial fibrillation, and the bradycardia component is a long pause that is followed by a junctional escape beat. Symptoms may include lightheadedness, fainting spells, fatigue, and palpitations.

The common faint is often associated with fear, the sight of blood (e.g., needle sticks), pain, emotional stress and brief premonitory signs and symptoms (e.g., nausea, abdominal discomfort, yawning, sweating, pallor, diminished hearing or blurred vision, a sense of lightheadedness *[graying out]*). It results from bradycardia and hypotension, caused by excessive vagal discharge (vasovagal, or neurocardiogenic, syncope), especially after prolonged upright posture (e.g., standing during religious services or in a crowded, hot room). Often there is a long antecedent history of similar episodes, especially during adolescence and young adulthood.

Figure 5-21. Causes of neurally mediated syncope: carotid sinus syncope occurring with **A.** shaving, **B.** wearing a tight collar, **C.** sudden turn of the head. Situational syncope, occurring during or immediately after **D.** urination or **E.** vigorous paroxysms of coughing, may result in a long "pause" (ECG strip, **bottom**) due to transient intense vagotonia with sinus node suppression.

Syncope in the setting of any GI symptoms (e.g., nausea, abdominal cramps, diarrhea) is likely to be vagal in origin.

Figure 5-22. Note: When evaluating the various degrees of AV block, keep in mind the following **mnemonic:** IF the "R" is far from "P," then you have

FIRST DEGREE. If longer, longer, longer, DROP! – then you have WENCKEBACH. If some "Ps" don't get through, then you have MOBITZ II. If "Ps" and "Qs" just don't agree, then you have THIRD DEGREE. (from the Heart Block Poem by the Princeton Surgical Group)

An arrhythmia that is caused by a delay or interruption of cardiac conduction is termed *heart block*. Heart blocks at the AV node:

A. *First-degree AV block*, where there is excessive delay at the AV node, resulting in a prolonged, constant PR interval > 0.20 sec.

B. *Mobitz type I second-degree AV block.* Note 3:2 *Wenckebach pattern*, i.e., PR interval gets progressively longer until P wave isn't conducted. The sequence is then repeated (*group beating*).

C. *Mobitz type II second-degree AV block.* Fixed PR interval with some non-premature P waves not conducted (dropped QRS beats, 3:2 block in this case).

D. *Third-degree (complete) AV block.* Varying PR intervals, i.e., atria and ventricles are contracting independently of each other, and the atrial rate is faster than the ventricular rate.

Bundle Branch Block

The characteristics of right and left bundle branch block were presented in **Chapter 2** in the discussion of analysis of the QRS complex.

Figure 5-23. 12-lead ECG tracing demonstrating the characteristic features of right bundle branch block. Note the QRS is wide (>0.12 sec), an rSR' pattern (so-called *rabbit ears*) is present in leads V1 and V2, and a wide S wave is seen in leads I, aVL and V6.

Figure 5-24. 12-lead ECG tracing demonstrating the characteristic features of left bundle branch block. Note the QRS is wide (>0.12 sec), monophasic (or notched, not shown) R waves are present in leads I, aVL and V6, the QRS is mostly negative in V1–V3, the ST segment is in the opposite direction of the QRS, and is elevated in leads V1–V3. These ST-T changes are secondary to the conduction defect.

An ECG abnormality should always be interpreted in the context of the "company it keeps." For example, right bundle branch block, although it may be seen in congenital heart disease (e.g., atrial septal defect) and conditions affecting the conduction system (e.g., sclerodegenerative disease), may not have a serious import if it appears as an isolated finding (congenital abnormality) in a young, otherwise healthy individual. It is not unusual to detect RBBB in patients with no other clinical evidence of heart disease. On the other hand, if RBBB develops in the setting of an acute MI, it often has significant prognostic importance.

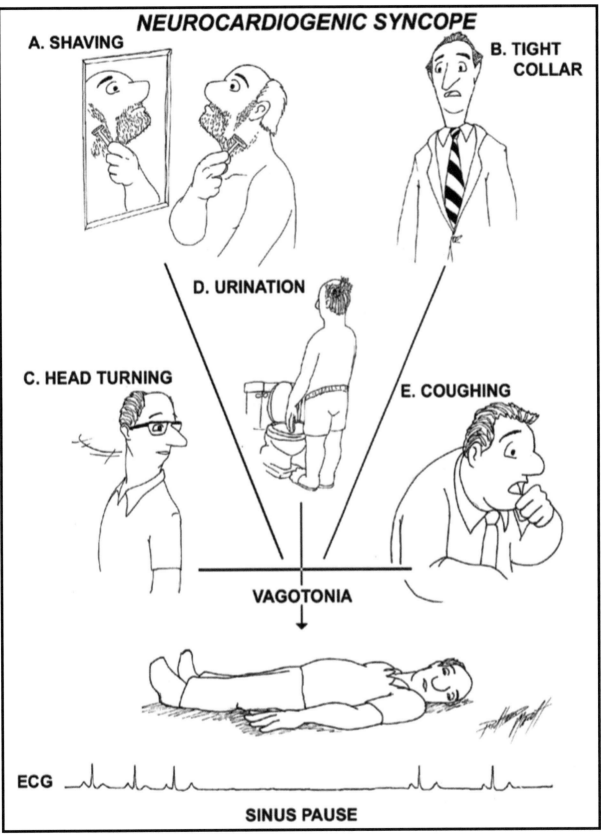

Fig. 5-21.

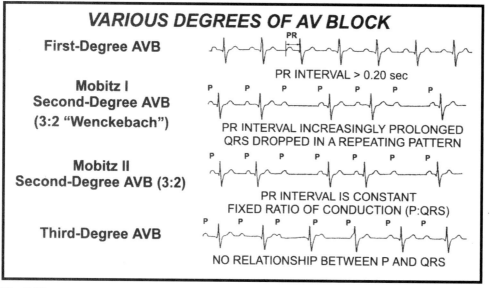

Fig. 5-22.

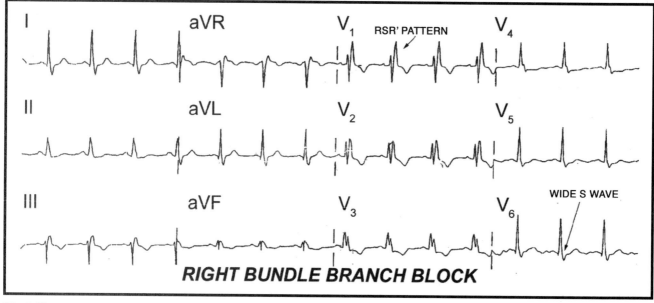

Fig. 5-23.

(**Note:** An inherited disorder [channelopathy] known as *Brugada syndrome* has been described in which RBBB with persistent ST segment elevation [coved or saddleback] in precordial leads V1–V2 is associated with the susceptibility to VT/VF and sudden cardiac death.) **(Figure 5-25)**

Figure 5-25. Conventional precordial ECG leads in a patient with the *Brugada syndrome*. Note the ST segment elevation in leads V1-V3 along with a right bundle branch morphology in lead V1. These patients may develop ventricular tachycardia, ventricular fibrillation, and sudden cardiac death.

In contrast, the new appearance of LBBB is decidedly more ominous than RBBB. LBBB is usually associated with organic heart disease and is only occasionally seen in normal subjects. It is associated with significantly reduced long-term survival, with 10-year survival rates as low as 50%. It is commonly associated with long-standing hypertension, CAD, dilated cardiomyopathy, calcific aortic valvular

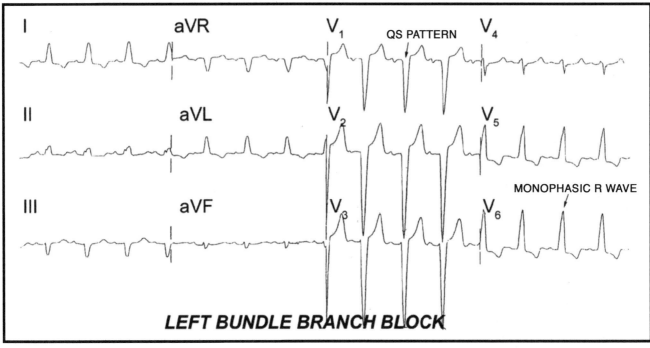

Fig. 5-24.

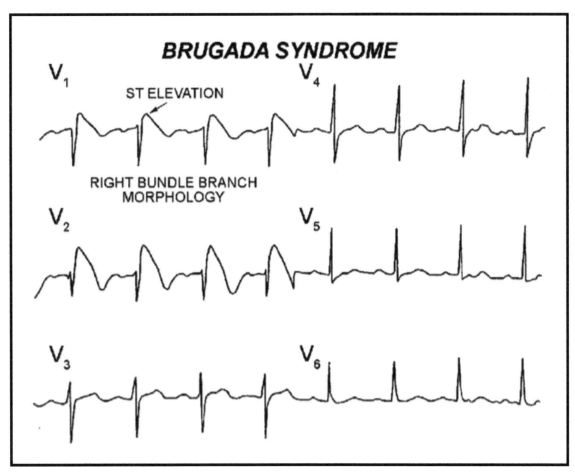

Fig. 5-25.

disease, and degenerative conduction system disease. LBBB may be the first clue to underlying heart muscle disease (e.g., cardiomyopathy). In the setting of symptoms highly consistent with myocardial ischemia, the presence of a new (or presumably new) LBBB on the ECG should raise the suspicion of acute MI with proximal occlusion of the LAD. In general, patients with CAD and LBBB often have a higher incidence of multivessel disease, LV systolic dysfunction, and a poorer prognosis.

Transient (intermittent) bundle branch block may also occur when the heart rate increases or decreases to a critical rate (rate-dependent block). The BBB resolves when the heart rate returns to baseline. Transient BBB is a manifestation of a diseased His-Purkinje system.

Fascicular Block

Fascicular blocks (also known as *hemiblocks*) represent disturbed conduction in either the anterior or posterior division, or fascicle, of the left bundle branch. The anterior fascicle is long and thin and has a single blood supply (LAD), which makes it more vulnerable to block than the posterior fascicle, which is short and thick and has a dual blood supply (LAD and right coronary artery).

Figure 5-26 illustrates the *hemiblock patterns* in the limb leads. The "anterior" papillary muscle of the left ventricle is above (rather than inferior) and lateral to the "posterior" papillary muscle, and the two divisions of the left bundle branch course towards their respective papillary muscles. If the anterior division is blocked (*left*

anterior hemiblock), initial forces are directed downwards and to the right (toward the posterior papillary muscle), inscribing a q wave in lead I and an r wave in lead II. The subsequent forces are directed mainly upwards and to the left (toward the anterior papillary muscle), inscribing an R wave in lead I and an S wave in lead II, producing a left axis deviation. In left posterior hemiblock, the opposite holds true. The initial forces spread upwards and to the left, inscribing an r in lead I and a q in lead II. Subsequent forces are directed downwards and to the right, inscribing an S wave in lead I and an R wave in lead II, producing a right axis deviation.

Although hemiblock can occur by itself, left anterior hemiblock is often (and left posterior hemiblock almost always) associated with RBBB (so-called *bifascicular block*). The combination of RBBB with both left anterior hemiblock and left posterior hemiblock is called *trifascicular block*. A word of caution: Although a prolonged PR interval in the presence of bifascicular block may, at times, be indicative of trifascicular block, such a pattern is more likely to indicate that the block is at the level of the AV node, rather than the third remaining fascicle. Hemiblock, like bundle branch block, is commonly caused by CAD. Other causes include cardiomyopathy, sclerodegenerative disease, and aortic valve calcification.

Block within the bundle branches or their divisions often precedes the development of complete heart block. The combination of RBBB and left anterior hemiblock is seen commonly, and AV conduction is dependent on the integrity of the posterior division of the left bundle. If progression of disease in the posterior division occurs, complete heart block can result.

Cardiac Pacemakers

When complete (third-degree) AV block, symptomatic second-degree AV block, sick sinus syndrome, or symptomatic bradycardia exist, a cardiac pacemaker may be required. A cardiac pacemaker is an electronic device that creates and transmits an electrical signal to the heart. It consists of an electronic pulse generator, a battery, and one or more electrodes (also called *leads*) that sense the electrical activity of the heart and deliver electrical impulses to the atria or ventricles or both when needed.

Pacemakers are described by a 4-letter code:

- The first letter refers to the chamber(s) *paced*, i.e., Atrial (A), Ventricular (V), or Dual (D).
- The second letter refers to the chamber(s) *sensed* (A, V, or D).
- The third letter refers to the pacemaker *mode*, i.e., Inhibited (I), Triggered (T), or Dual (D).

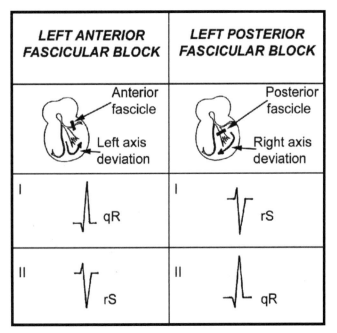

LEFT ANTERIOR FASCICULAR BLOCK	LEFT POSTERIOR FASCICULAR BLOCK
Anterior fascicle / Left axis deviation	Posterior fascicle / Right axis deviation
I ⊣↓⊢ qR	I ⊣↓⊢ rS
II ⊣↓⊢ rS	II ⊣↓⊢ qR

Fig. 5-26.

- The fourth letter refers to *programmable functions*. The letter R = rate responsiveness, which denotes that the device has a sensor that increases the pacing rate in response to a perceived physiologic requirement.

Most pacemaker programming results in inhibition of the pacemaker when the intrinsic rate is higher than the lower pacing rate.

A typical *single-chamber* demand (backup) pacemaker is a VVI, which paces in the right ventricle, senses in the ventricle, and inhibits ventricular pacing if there is a sensed QRS. A typical *dual-chamber* pacemaker is the DDDR, which paces and senses both the right atrium and right ventricle, and inhibits and triggers a paced response. Both pacemaker types are rate-responsive to exercise (by sensing body motion or respiratory rate). A pacemaker that senses and paces in both chambers is the most physiologic approach to pacing patients who remain in sinus rhythm. Dual chamber (AV sequential) pacing is most useful for individuals with LV systolic or, perhaps more importantly, diastolic dysfunction since they preserve *atrial kick*. (Atrial contraction contributes as much as 30% to cardiac output.)

For many years, most cardiac pacing was ventricular in either the fixed-rate or demand (standby) mode. Present pacemaker technology has made early fixed-rate pacemakers obsolete. Only demand-type pacemakers are in current use. VVI or VVIR (ventricular leads only) pacing is particularly appropriate when there is chronic atrial fibrillation (i.e., no *atrial kick*) and when there is a short life expectancy and low risk for *pacemaker syndrome* (fatigue, weakness, dyspnea, diminished exercise tolerance, even to the point of CHF, lightheadedness). Patients with VVI pacemakers, however, may develop pacemaker syndrome due to loss of AV synchrony, resulting in a drop in cardiac output, especially in stiff, noncompliant ventricles (e.g., CAD, hypertension, valvular AS, HOCM).

Figure 5-27. Left. In a single chamber (ventricular) demand (VVI) pacemaker, 1 pacing lead is implanted in the apex of the right ventricle. **Right**. Note the drop in BP (second tracing from the top) during ventricular paced beats due to loss of *atrial kick*.

Once it is evident that a pacemaker is present, you can identify the chambers that are sensed and paced, and whether the pacemaker is functioning properly. When the cardiac rhythm is initiated by the impulse from an artificial pacemaker, pacing spikes can usually be detected on an ECG as positively or negatively directed vertical lines. Clues to ventricular paced rhythm include a wide QRS with a LBBB pattern and left axis deviation (since pacing originates from the RV apex).

A normally functioning dual chamber (AV sequential) pacemaker is associated with four different rhythms, depending on the heart's intrinsic activity:

1. Complete inhibition (pacing spikes are absent). The pacemaker senses intrinsic impulses from the atria and ventricles.
2. Atrial pacing with conduction (paced P waves and intrinsic QRS complexes). Atrial pacing occurs when the intrinsic atrial rate falls below the programmed rate.
3. Atrial sensing and ventricular pacing (intrinsic P waves and paced QRS complexes). The pacemaker senses a native atrial impulse that inhibits the device from firing; however, the impulse fails to conduct to the ventricles, which results in a paced QRS complex.
4. AV sequential pacing (paced P waves and paced QRS complexes). Atrial and ventricular pacing occurs as conduction depends entirely on the pacemaker.

Figure 5-28. Left. In a dual chamber (AV sequential) pacemaker, 2 pacing leads are implanted (1 in the apex

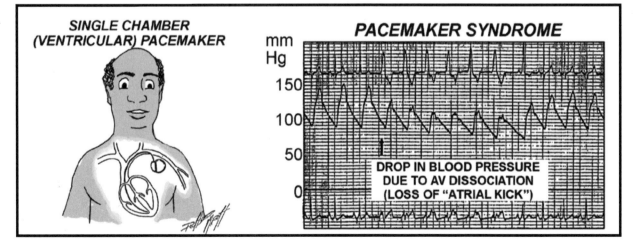

Fig. 5-27.

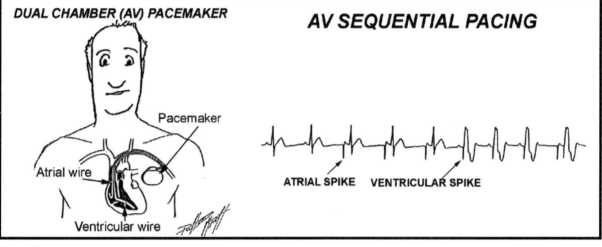

Fig. 5-28.

of the right ventricle and 1 in the right atrium). This is the most common type of implanted pacemaker. An AV sequential pacemaker paces either the atria, the ventricles, or both sequentially when spontaneous electrical activity is absent.

Right. ECG tracing demonstrating AV sequential pacing with mode switching. Note the atrial and ventricular pacemaker spikes that precede the P wave and QRS complex. Also note the wide QRS complex that results from direct activation of the ventricular myocardium. In the last complex, the atrial electrode paces the atrium and, after a programmed delay, signals the ventricular electrode to pace the ventricle (AV sequential pacing). If the patient's intrinsic sinus rate is faster than the programmed atrial pacing rate, the pacemaker switches to a P triggered mode (6th-8th complexes). If the patient's AV conduction resumes and the sinus rate is fast enough, both the atrial and ventricular pacing will be inhibited (1st and 2nd complexes). If the AV conduction becomes normal, but the sinus rate is not fast enough, the pacemaker switches to an atrial pacing mode (3rd-5th complexes).

Early permanent pacemakers were powered by mercury zinc batteries. These have been replaced by lithium batteries, which have improved longevity (4-10 years). The insertion of a permanent pacemaker is frequently lifesaving and improves the quality of life. Although complications of permanent pacing are uncommon, they may occur. These include malfunction due to lead displacement or fracture.

Pacemaker malfunction may include

- *Failure to pace* (indicated by absence of pacemaker spikes when there is an indication for pacing)
- *Failure to capture* (indicated by a pacemaker spike without the appropriate atrial or ventricular response, i.e., a spike without a P wave or QRS complex)
- *Undersensing* or *failure to sense* (indicated by a pacemaker spike that fires inappropriately when intrinsic electrical activity is already present – a spike may appear in the middle or after native P waves and QRS complexes)
- *Oversensing* (indicated by a paced beat that appears later than expected due to inappropriate sensing of the wrong electrical signal, e.g., pectoral muscle movements (myopotentials)

Figure 5-29. Pacemaker malfunction. **A.** Failure to pace – no paced beat when there should be one. **B.** Failure to capture – a pacer spike but no QRS complex. **C.** Failure to sense – pacer spikes fire anywhere, with one falling on a T wave *(R on T phenomenon)* causing *torsades de pointes*. **D.** Oversensing – paced beat appears later than it should because pectoral myopotentials are sensed and mistaken for QRS complexes.

Figure 5-30. Biventricular pacing is also known as *cardiac resynchronization therapy (CRT)*. It is used in the management of heart failure with ventricular dyssynchrony, which may cause a prolonged QRS complex due to slowing of intraventricular conduction. In a biventricular pacemaker, in addition to pacing leads in the right atrium and right ventricles, a third pacing lead is advanced from the coronary sinus to the lateral wall of the left ventricle (allows pacing of the LV simultaneously with the RV and helps resynchronize cardiac activation, thereby improving LV function). Cardiac resynchronization therapy creates a fusion pattern between the LV pacing site and the RV pacing site. Usually there is a narrow RBBB-like QRS complex (tall R wave in lead V1) that is distinctly different from pacing at the RV apex alone.

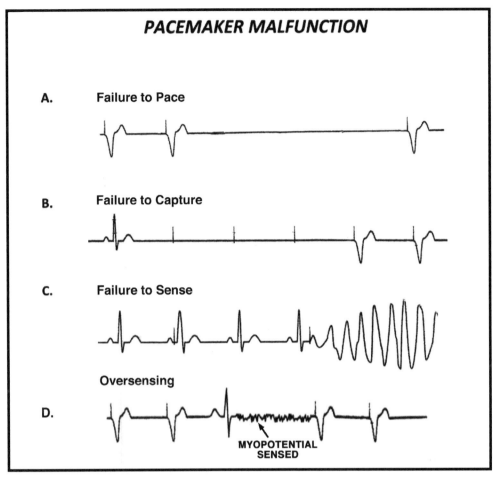

Fig. 5-29.

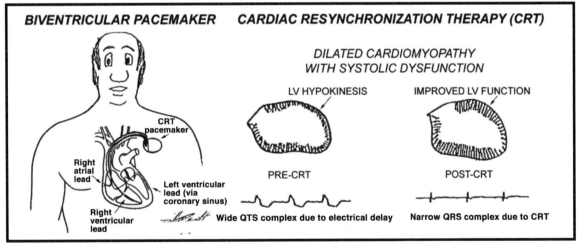

Fig. 5-30.

Most patients eligible for CRT also meet the criteria for an implantable cardioverter defibrillator (ICD) and receive a combined device. The ICD is capable of delivering shocks to the heart to interrupt a life-threatening run of VT or VF.

Figure 5-31. Left. Implantable cardioverter defibrillator (ICD); early (left) and contemporary (right) models. Note that the early ICD system used epicardial patch electrodes for defibrillation and epicardial leads for rate sensing.

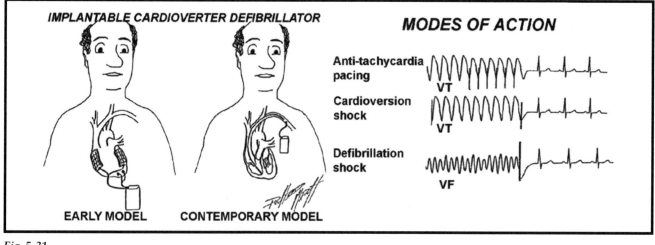

Fig. 5-31.

Right. The current model has leads with both sensing and defibrillating function and can sense VT, with antitachycardia pacing and/or shocks. If an episode of VT occurs, the ICD will normally begin by trying to overdrive pace the arrhythmia to terminate it. If that fails, the device will usually go on to deliver a shock. If VF is detected, a shock is delivered as first-line treatment.

* * *

Pearls:

- The most common "cause of a pause" is a blocked PAC.

- A narrow-complex supraventricular tachycardia (SVT) that has a regular heart rate of 150 beats/min is atrial flutter with 2:1 AV block, until proven otherwise.

- An irregularly irregular rhythm in a patient with COPD is more commonly *multifocal atrial tachycardia* (MAT) than atrial fibrillation. MAT is an irregular fast rhythm defined by the presence of 3 or more P waves of varying morphologies. It may also be caused by hypokalemia or hypomagnesemia. MAT occurs most commonly in chronic lung disease but is also seen in patients with severe metabolic abnormalities or sepsis.

- Compare the ECG with previous tracings. Prior tracings may reveal ectopic complexes (PACs, PVCs), a prolonged QT interval, pre-existing bundle branch block, or WPW syndrome, and provide clues to the origin of the current arrhythmia.

- If there is an abrupt onset and termination of a regular narrow complex tachycardia, think of AVNRT.

- Wide complex tachycardia in the setting of structural heart disease (e.g., acute MI, dilated cardiomyopathy) is VT until proven otherwise.

- If there is a short PR interval and delta wave on a previous ECG, consider WPW as the possible reason for a "bizarre" tachyarrhythmia.

- In patients with atrial fibrillation, an excessively fast ventricular response (>250 beats/min) may be a clue to WPW syndrome and the presence of an accessory pathway (and the need to avoid digoxin, beta blockers, and calcium channel blockers, since any drug that blocks the AV node can accelerate the rhythm and precipitate VF).

- All narrow complex rhythms are supraventricular in origin, but not all supraventricular rhythms have a narrow complex.

- All rhythms that begin in the ventricle have a wide QRS complex, but not all wide rhythms are ventricular in origin.

- All of the following are clues favoring the diagnosis of VT over SVT with aberrancy: the presence of AV dissociation, extremely wide QRS complexes with morphology not typical of RBBB or LBBB, QRS concordance (all QRS complexes in the same direction in V1-V6), and fusion (or capture) beats in the setting of underlying heart disease (especially prior MI).

- Atrial fibrillation, MAT, and atrial flutter produce irregularly irregular QRS complexes. However, with MAT, P waves of 3 or more differing morphologies precede the QRS complexes. With atrial flutter, flutter waves *(sawtooth pattern)* often are visible between the QRS complexes.

- Always keep in mind that when P waves are halfway between QRS complexes, there may be another P wave hiding in or near the QRS complex, and the rhythm represents some variety of SVT with 2:1 conduction. If the rate is >150 beats/min, think of atrial flutter with 2:1 block.

- If a regular tachycardia is present, observe the response to vagal maneuvers. SVT may revert back to NSR; VT generally will not.
- If on examining a *stable* patient, you detect a regular sinus rhythm with a slow ventricular rate (i.e., sinus bradycardia in the 50's or 60's), think of two things: 1) the patient is a well-trained athlete or is physically conditioned (vagal tone), or 2) the patient might be taking a rate-slowing medication (e.g., beta blocker, calcium channel blocker, amiodarone, clonidine, lithium). An *unstable* patient (e.g., acute inferior MI), on the other hand, may also have a slow heart rate. Keep in mind that timolol eye drops (a beta blocker) in the elderly may result in sufficient systemic absorption to slow the sinus node or unmask sinus node dysfunction. The medications your patient is receiving must always be considered when evaluating heart rate.

- The onset of AV conduction system disease (first-, second-, or third-degree AV block) in a young patient with a flu-like illness and a rash should raise the suspicion of *Lyme disease*, the leading tick-borne disease in the United States (caused by Borrelia burgdorferi, a spirochetal organism transmitted by the bite of the deer tick). Heart block usually resolves following treatment with antibiotics.

* * *

6

Miscellaneous ECG Patterns

A few miscellaneous clinical conditions that are associated with characteristic ECG changes warrant discussion. The differential diagnosis of ST segment elevation frequently presents a diagnostic challenge in patients who present with chest pain.

Pericarditis

Acute pericarditis (inflammation of the pericardium) can cause changes on the ECG that mimic ischemia or infarction.

Most cases of pericarditis are idiopathic, and presumed to be viral. Pericarditis may also result from malignancy, connective tissue disease, chest trauma, cardiac surgery, certain medications (e.g., hydralazine,

procainamide), end-stage renal disease, and other causes of inflammation.

The ST segment elevations with acute MI are typically convex and localized to the area of the infarct. In contrast, the ST elevations with pericarditis are usually concave and diffuse, and do not follow the pattern of blood supply. As a rule, these ST elevations are not accompanied by reciprocal depressions of the ST segment in the other leads. These ST elevations are due to an epicardial current of injury produced by the pericardial inflammatory process.

Figure 6-1. Typical 12-lead ECG tracing in a patient with acute pericarditis. Diffuse concave upward (valley-like) ST segment elevation (in all leads except aVR and V1) along with PR segment depression and

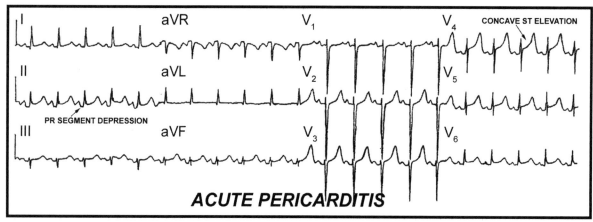

Fig. 6-1.

downsloping of the TP segment (so-called *Spodick's sign*),may provide helpful clues to the diagnosis of *pericarditis*. T wave inversions typically do not appear until ST segment elevations have resolved. Eventually the T waves return to the normal upright position.

Pericardial effusion may also be seen in patients with pericarditis. The most common ECG sign of pericardial effusion is low voltage of the QRS complexes. Total electrical alternans of the P, QRS and T waves may also be seen, and is virtually pathognomonic of cardiac tamponade, often due to metastatic cancer.

Figure 6-2. Low voltage and total *electrical alternans* (alternating ECG complex heights) of the P, QRS, and T waves (due to the swinging motion of the heart) strengthens the clinical suspicion of *pericardial effusion with tamponade*, as seen in precordial leads V2-V4 in this 12-lead ECG.

Early Repolarization

Early repolarization is an ECG pattern of widespread ST segment elevation. The ST segment elevations seen with early repolarization are stable and do not undergo the evolutionary sequence seen with acute MI or pericarditis.

Figure 6-3. In *early repolarization* in healthy, asymptomatic, young individuals, concave upward ST segment elevation (most often seen in the precordial

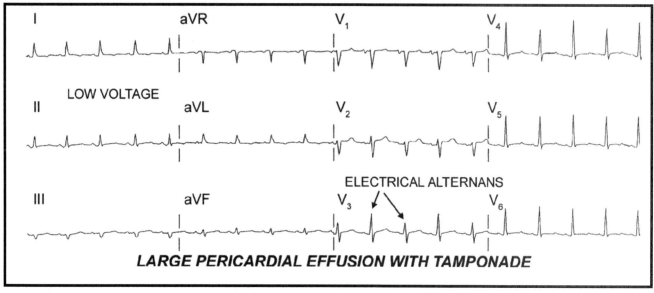

Fig. 6-2.

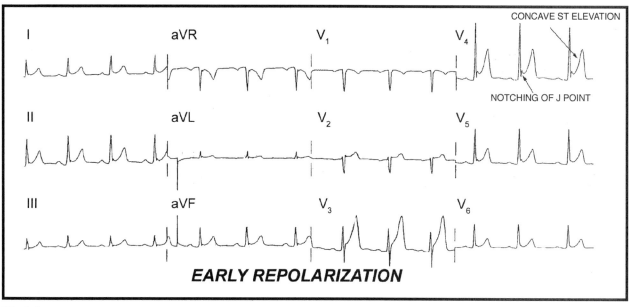

Fig. 6-3.

leads) along with notching of the J point (the junction of QRS with the beginning of the ST segment) can mimic acute MI or pericarditis. This is generally a "benign" variant, especially in African-American males and trained athletes, as seen in this 12-lead ECG. Notching in the J point (lead V4) and upward concavity *(smile-like)* of the ST segment favor early repolarization pattern *(fishhook appearance)*. Pericarditis can be distinguished from early repolarization by the ratio of the ST elevation to the T wave. If the ST elevation is < 1/4 of the T wave amplitude, then early repolarization is present. Furthermore, the ST elevation from early repolarization resolves with exercise, while that of pericarditis does not.

Note: A "malignant" variant of early repolarization has been described in which notching of the J point in the inferolateral leads may be associated with an increased risk of VF, but the absolute risk is low.

Early repolarization can present a diagnostic challenge because it may mimic an acute MI or pericarditis. These conditions can be distinguished from each other with the recognition of their characteristic ECG findings summarized in **Figure 6-4**.

Hypothermia

A convex elevation of the J point (J wave or *Osborn wave*) may also be seen with profound *hypothermia* (below 33° C). The height of the Osborn (J) wave is proportional to the degree of hypothermia and is thought to result from repolarization abnormalities of the ventricle (**Figure 2-11L**).

Figure 6-5. Osborn (J) waves in hypothermia. The height of the J wave is proportional to the degree of hypothermia. Patients with hypothermia may also

	FIGURE 6-4 COMPARISON OF ECG FINDINGS IN ACUTE MYOCARDIAL INFARCTION, PERICARDITIS, AND EARLY REPOLARIZATION		
ECG FINDINGS	**ACUTE MYOCARDIAL INFARCTION**	**ACUTE PERICARDITIS**	**EARLY REPOLARIZATION**
ST segment elevation	Convex upward	Concave upward	Concave upward
Q wave	Present	Absent	Absent
Reciprocal ST segment changes	Present	Absent	Absent
Location of ST segment elevation	Area of involved myocardium	Limb and chest leads	Limb and chest leads
PR segment depression	Absent	Present	Absent

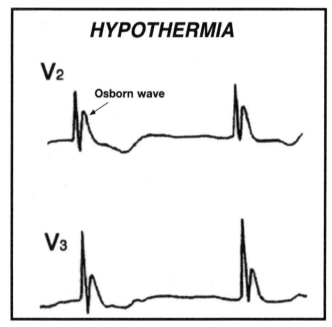

Fig. 6-5.

exhibit other ECG abnormalities, including AV block, atrial fibrillation, wide QRS complexes, prolonged QT interval, ventricular arrhythmias, and asystole.

Left Ventricular Aneurysm

Left ventricular aneurysms typically occur in patients who have had a large anterior wall MI resulting from persistent total occlusion of the proximal portion of the poorly collateralized left anterior descending coronary artery. They can lead to heart failure, ventricular arrhythmias, and embolic events (due to mural thrombus formation). LV aneurysms may be associated with ST segment elevations that persist weeks to months after an acute MI.

Figure 6-6. LV aneurysm. This patient had a previous anterior MI. Persistence of *both* Q waves and ST segment elevation in the anterior leads several weeks or more after an MI may provide a clue to an LV aneurysm.

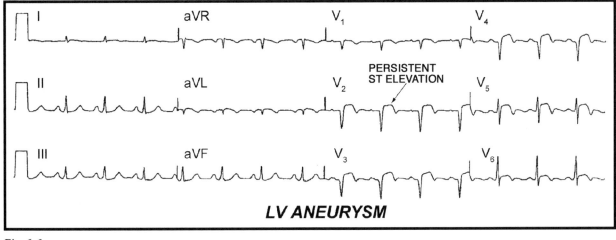

Fig. 6-6.

Mimics of Myocardial Ischemia and Infarction

There are many causes of ST segment and T wave abnormalities that can mimic those of ischemia (e.g., LV hypertrophy and electrolyte, metabolic, and drug-induced effects). Other clinical conditions, e.g., Takotsubo (stress) cardiomyopathy, as well as Brugada syndrome and arrhythmogenic RV cardiomyopathy, inherited disorders associated with ventricular arrhythmias and sudden cardiac death, can also produce ST segment elevation on the ECG (see **Figures 5-25 and 7-6**). These are known as "infarct imposters." The clinician should also be aware of the wide spectrum of normal variations, especially pertaining to repolarization patterns, and not falsely label a healthy patient as having heart disease on the basis of a non-specific finding (e.g., persistent juvenile pattern T wave inversion, a common normal variant), which may be of no significance and lead to unnecessary anxiety and potential harm. ST and T wave changes are the most common and sensitive of the ECG abnormalities but are also the least specific.

Remember that an "abnormal-looking" ECG does not necessarily mean that the patient has CAD or even an abnormal heart. Mimics of an MI, age indeterminate, include:

- Incorrect chest lead placement
- Normal variant (e.g., QS pattern in leads V1 and V2 even with correct lead placement)

- LV hypertrophy with poor R wave progression in leads V1-V3, mimicking anteroseptal MI
- Incomplete LBBB
- Cor pulmonale secondary to COPD with poor R wave progression or a QS pattern in the precordial leads
- WPW syndrome with pseudo-Q waves mimicking anterior or inferior MI (see **Figures 3-20** and **3-21**).
- HOCM with Q waves in the inferolateral leads
- Involvement of the heart by amyloid, sarcoidosis, scleroderma, neoplasm, or neuromuscular disease
- A misdiagnosis of an old anteroseptal MI (due to "poor R wave progression") can be made in a patient with a long asthenic chest build, and a "teardrop" heart. Electrode placement, even though in the correct interspace, is the culprit. You should place the chest leads one or two interspaces lower, and the normal progression of R wave (rather than slow) may result.

In addition, don't be disappointed when an ECG tracing is returned with an interpretation of "non-specific ST-T changes." To suggest that such changes always represent "ischemia" significantly overstates the accuracy of the test and can lead to serious consequences. For example, T wave inversions in leads V1-V3 are more likely to represent a normal variant in a healthy young female (*juvenile T wave pattern*) than the same findings in a middle-aged or older male with chest discomfort and risk factors, where it may represent a clue to underlying CAD.

7

Pearls and Pitfalls In ECG Interpretation

When interpreted correctly, the 12-lead ECG remains a highly useful clinical tool in the evaluation of the patient with known or suspected heart disease. Regrettably, many anxious and frightened but otherwise healthy individuals today are carrying the stigma of "false" heart disease, along with its attendant and often tragic consequences resulting from an incorrect diagnosis due to misinterpretation of the patient's ECG. This chapter will provide an overview of some of the most common errors in ECG interpretation made in everyday clinical practice. A practical approach to differentiating normal (*physiologic*) from abnormal (*pathologic*) ECG findings in the well-trained athlete will also be discussed.

Misinterpretation of ECG Findings

Many patients with chest pain of non-cardiac origin also happen to have a so-called *abnormal ECG*. Over-interpretation of insignificant changes on the ECG (e.g., nonspecific ST-T wave abnormalities) may falsely label healthy patients as having heart disease.

Figure 7-1. 12-lead ECG tracing showing *poor R wave progression*. The patient has no underlying heart disease. In a normal heart, the R waves should become gradually taller from leads V1-V6, with the R/S ratio >1 by lead V4. If the R waves remain small in leads V1-V3 (or V4), *poor R wave progression* is said to be present. This may be caused by an anteroseptal MI, COPD, LV hypertrophy, dilated cardiomyopathy, misplaced chest leads, clockwise rotation of the heart or it may represent a normal variant.

In childhood, the precordial T waves are commonly inverted in leads V1-V3, and their continued presence in young adults (*persistent juvenile pattern*) is a common normal variant.

Figure 7-2. ECG tracing in a young marathon runner. Note the T wave may normally be inverted in the precordial leads (*juvenile T wave pattern*).

Poor technique can lead to misinterpretation of the ECG, wasted investigations, and mismanagement of the patient. Reversal of the arm leads, if not recognized, may lead to a spurious diagnosis of lateral wall MI.

Figure 7-3. 12-lead ECG tracing in a young asymptomatic technology student practicing ECG technique. This tracing represents an example of misplaced leads, i.e., right and left arm limb lead reversal. Note the negative P wave, QRS and T wave in lead I, which may mimic dextrocardia. However, in contrast to dextrocardia, there is normal R wave progression in the precordial leads.

Incorrect placement of the precordial leads may also lead to a false diagnosis of MI. In addition, QRS abnormalities (e.g., as may occur in patients with WPW syndrome) may also be misdiagnosed as an MI. Patient-related technical factors (e.g., muscle tremors and movement, as seen in Parkinson's disease) may create artifacts that result in an incorrect diagnosis of arrhythmias (e.g., atrial flutter/fibrillation, VT/VF), which may lead to unnecessary interventions and treatment.

Figure 7-4. A motion artifact simulating ventricular tachycardia. This tracing "caught the attention" of the

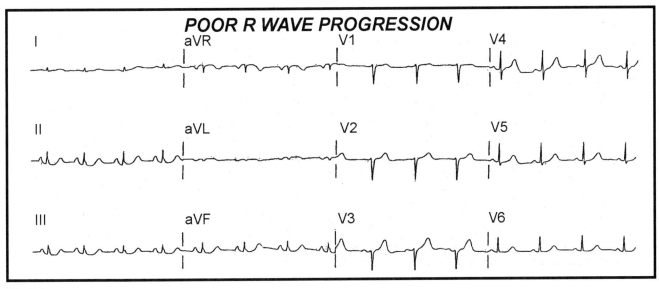

Fig. 7-1.

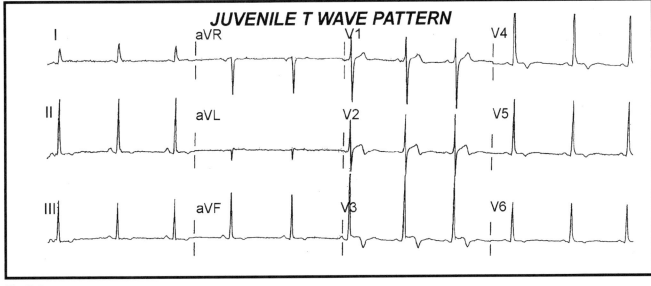

Fig. 7-2.

cath lab staff during a routine diagnostic study. Note the presence of the same movement artifact disturbing the arterial pulse tracing. Misinterpretation of ECG artifacts may result in unnecessary therapeutic intervention (e.g., antiarrhythmic drugs, implantation of an ICD).

Limitations of Computer ECG Analysis

The over-reliance on *computer interpretation of ECGs* nowadays has also created a significant source of confusion. A computer interpretation of "normal ECG" is often, but not always, correct. Over-diagnosis of normal or insignificant findings is not unusual, and the astute clinician needs to be aware of these "variants" of normal. The computer makes routine measurement (e.g., heart rate, QRS duration, and electrical axis) accurately and quickly. However, the computer has difficulty separating small waves from a noisy baseline, often resulting from artifacts, and is often incorrect in detecting arrhythmias, e.g., atrial fibrillation. These misdiagnoses occur because the computer has difficulty in identifying low amplitude P waves, especially if they are hidden in T waves or baseline skeletal muscle artifact. The computer may overcall a normal ECG as one showing a previous myocardial infarction. Poor R wave progression is frequently overcalled as a previous

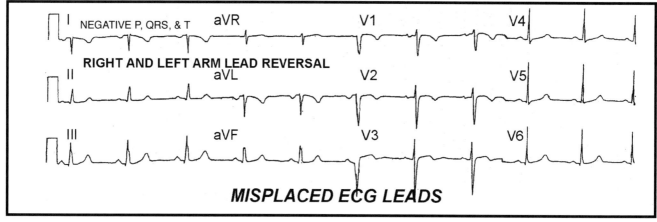

Fig. 7-3.

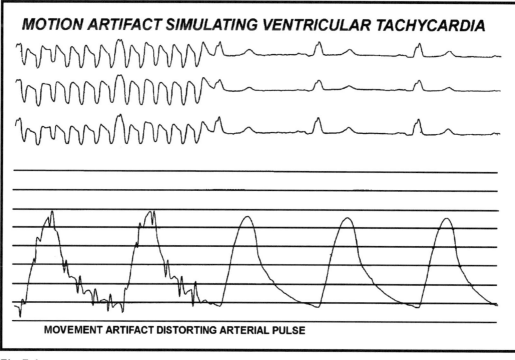

Fig. 7-4.

anteroseptal MI. Similarly, an isolated Q wave in lead III is often overcalled as an old inferior wall MI. All ST elevation tends to be diagnosed as an acute STEMI, even when due to pericarditis, or even more disturbingly, when physiological (due to early repolarization). These errors are common and can lead to serious errors in management. For example, the misdiagnosis of atrial fibrillation can lead to unnecessary anticoagulation and/or the use of antiarrhythmic agents. The incorrect diagnosis of MI can lead to unnecessary coronary angiography or fibrinolysis.

Misleading clues may also arise from a pacemaker. Pacemaker spikes may be quite small, and if they are missed, a ventricular rhythm, MI, or LBBB can be erroneously diagnosed.

Virtually every variety of supraventricular and ventricular tachy/brady arrhythmias has been mimicked and consequently misdiagnosed as a result of artifacts registered during ambulatory ECG (Holter) monitoring (e.g., resulting from a loose or mechanical "stimulation" of an electrode, or failure of the battery or motor of the recorder, causing slowing of the tape speed).

Figure 7-5. An example of artifact on Holter monitor recording simulating sinus arrest. Note the loss of the U wave in the last beat on the upper strip. (Courtesy of Dr. Bernard D. Kosowsky). The main cause of pseudo sinus arrest is disconnection of an electrode or, less commonly, fracture of a cable. Misinterpretation of these artifacts may lead to unnecessary pacemaker insertion.

Exercise ECG stress testing may also yield "false positive" results that may be erroneously diagnosed as CAD. According to *Bayes theorem*, the predictive value of a diagnostic test is influenced by the pre-test likelihood of the disease in the population being tested. In the individual with a low pre-test probability of having CAD, a positive test has a high likelihood of being "falsely positive" (i.e., not due to myocardial ischemia). This may occur especially in young asymptomatic females (in whom the likelihood of CAD is very low), or in the setting of hyperventilation or when nonspecific ST-T abnormalities on the resting ECG are present. False positive exercise-induced ST segment changes are commonly seen with:

- Preexisting ST segment depression >1 mm at rest
- Pressure overload (e.g., hypertension, valvular aortic stenosis, hypertrophic cardiomyopathy)
- Electrolyte imbalance (e.g., hypokalemia)
- Drugs (e.g., digitalis)
- Women with mitral valve prolapse
- Premenopausal women with ST segment changes

- LV hypertrophy with *strain pattern*
- Left bundle branch block (LBBB)
- Paced ventricular rhythm
- Preexcitation (WPW) syndrome
- Hyperventilation

Since false positive tests often exceed true positives, leading to much patient anxiety and disability, exercise testing of asymptomatic individuals should be performed only for those at high risk (e.g., strong family history of premature CAD, or hyperlipidemia) or those with occupations that place them or others at special risk (e.g., airline pilots). Nuclear imaging may further confuse the clinician by demonstrating perfusion defects due to attenuation artifacts (e.g., breast tissue, elevated diaphragm, obesity) when, in fact, no defect exists.

The Athlete's Heart

Clinical evaluation of the well-trained athlete may present a challenge. ECG findings that at first appear "abnormal" are not uncommon in healthy young athletes. You should be aware that intensive physical training may alter the cardiovascular system in such a way as to create pseudo-abnormal findings (the *athletic heart syndrome*).

There are many variations of heart rate, rhythm, conduction, and alteration of both depolarization and

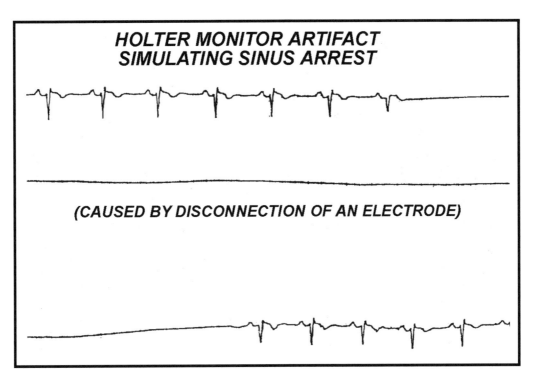

Fig. 7-5.

repolarization that are considered to be within the range of "normal" in the well-trained athlete. Common "normal" resting ECG and ambulatory (Holter) ECG findings in the athlete include:

- Sinus bradycardia, sinus arrhythmia, and sinus pauses
- First-degree AV block
- Second-degree AV block of the Wenckebach type (from enhanced vagal tone)
- AV junctional escape rhythm
- Ectopic supraventricular and ventricular beats
- Vertical axis
- Right axis deviation
- Incomplete RBBB
- LV hypertrophy
- Minor ST-T wave changes
- *Pseudo* anterolateral wall ischemia
- Early repolarization changes

As a rule, ST-T wave changes on the resting ECG in athletes tend to normalize during exercise. Stress testing, therefore, may help avoid the misdiagnosis of CAD. To avoid over-interpretation and inappropriate diagnosis of heart disease in these special individuals, the range of reported physiologic changes in the cardiovascular system in the athlete should be understood and correctly recognized.

The distinction between the athlete's heart and cardiac disease has important implications. The diagnosis of heart disease in an athlete may disqualify him or her from participation in competition. However, with certain cardiac conditions, participation in competitive athletics carries the risk for sudden death. Many of the conditions responsible for sudden cardiac death in the athlete can be suspected and even diagnosed by means of a careful and thoughtful interpretation of the ECG (**Figure 7-6**).

Figure 7-6. ECG markers of sudden cardiac death. Specific abnormalities to look for include

A. marked LV hypertrophy (*HOCM*)
B. ST segment–T wave changes (*CAD*), including ST depression and/or T wave inversion (TWI) as in unstable angina (UA) or non STEMI, and ST elevation in STEMI
C. LBBB (*dilated cardiomyopathy*)
D. prolonged QT interval (*long QT syndrome*) with its attendant risk of polymorphic VT (*torsades de pointes*)
E. short PR interval and delta wave (*WPW syndrome*)
F. RBBB morphology with ST elevation in precordial leads V1-V2 (*Brugada syndrome*)
G. incomplete RBBB with a terminal notch in the QRS (*epsilon wave*) and T wave inversion in V1-V3 (*arrhythmogenic RV dysplasia/cardiomyopathy*)

H. Ventricular arrhythmias (e.g. ventricular tachycardia), which can also occur as a result of blunt chest wall trauma (commotio cordis), even in the absence of underlying heart disease.

While controversy surrounds the routine use of ECG as part of the preparticipation cardiovascular screening of athletes (due to the low prevalence of disease and high rate of false positive findings), the American Heart Association considers a targeted history and physical examination, designed to identify those conditions known to cause sudden cardiac death, to be the most practical and cost-effective approach. If any cardiovascular abnormality is detected or suspected on the initial evaluation, further testing can be obtained on an individual basis as needed.

Iatrogenic Heart Disease

The diagnostic process should always consider the possibility of a technical error (even considering the possibility of the wrong patient). It is important to check the name and date to be sure that it is the correct patient's ECG report. Seasoned consultants cannot always erase the fear that has been engendered by an initial "false" diagnosis of heart disease. Many so-called *cardiac cripples* who have no disabling cardiac disease, but who suffer from irreversible cardiac neuroses, practitioner-induced, are "limping" their way through life maimed as a result of a wrong diagnosis or careless statement about their hearts (*iatrogenic heart disease*).

Some heart disease terms should be avoided in the presence of patients or, if used, explained properly. For example, when the ECG term *block* is used (e.g., heart block, left or right bundle branch block, hemiblock), it is important to tell the patient that this is an electrical term and does not connote blockage of blood in the heart or circulation. Classifying a healthy patient as one with heart disease based on falsely positive ECG findings can cause much psychological harm and may lead to risks from unnecessary or inappropriate therapy. You should ask your patient to relate his or her perception of their problem to you in order to clear up any misperceptions regarding their condition.

* * *

Pearls:

- The ECG is the test of first choice for patients presenting with chest pain, syncope, or dizziness.
- The ECG is useful as a baseline in the initial assessment of patients with known cardiovascular disease and/or dysfunction. The ECG is also useful as part of the preoperative evaluation in patients

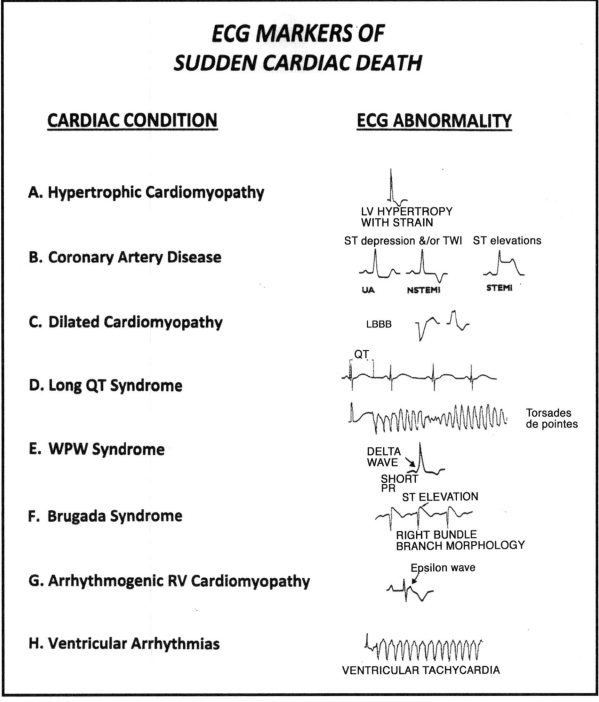

ECG MARKERS OF SUDDEN CARDIAC DEATH

CARDIAC CONDITION

A. Hypertrophic Cardiomyopathy

B. Coronary Artery Disease

C. Dilated Cardiomyopathy

D. Long QT Syndrome

E. WPW Syndrome

F. Brugada Syndrome

G. Arrhythmogenic RV Cardiomyopathy

H. Ventricular Arrhythmias

ECG ABNORMALITY

LV HYPERTROPY WITH STRAIN

ST depression &/or TWI   ST elevations

UA   NSTEMI   STEMI

LBBB

QT

Torsades de pointes

DELTA WAVE
SHORT PR

ST ELEVATION

RIGHT BUNDLE BRANCH MORPHOLOGY

Epsilon wave

VENTRICULAR TACHYCARDIA

Fig. 7-6.

>40 years of age, and in any patient with risk factors for CAD and/or known or suspected heart disease who are undergoing cardiac or noncardiac surgery (especially if a major operation, associated with large fluid shifts, or aortic or peripheral vascular surgery).

- The routine resting ECG (and even the exercise ECG) has significant limitations as a screening test in asymptomatic patients due to the high false positive and false negative rates.

- Although the presence of ST-T changes during episodes of chest pain is very helpful in diagnosing myocardial ischemia, the absence of such ECG findings does not exclude ischemic chest pain.

- Serial ECGs may be helpful in certain conditions (e.g., evolving acute MI). Serial ECGs permit evaluation of the response to treatment (e.g., thrombolytic therapy for acute MI) and of progression, remission or persistence of any abnormality noted on the baseline tracing.

- The ECG is an imprecise tool. A patient may have serious heart disease with little abnormality on the ECG, or no detectable heart disease, but an abnormal tracing.

- Don't over-interpret the ECG. The range of normal is wide, and there is considerable overlap between normal and abnormal.

- Before interpreting the ECG, make sure it has been taken correctly. Beware of technician errors (e.g., misplaced electrodes, lead reversal). Typically there should be a negative QRS complex in lead aVR. If there is not, suspect incorrect lead placement or dextrocardia. Always check for technical quality of the recording and calibration of the ECG machine. Keep on the lookout for baseline artifact (e.g., from disposable electrodes without proper skin preparation). Beware of patient movement and tremor (e.g., Parkinson's disease).

- To successfully interpret ECGs, have a systematic and logical approach. That is, assess heart rate and rhythm, P wave, QRS complex, ST and T wave, PR interval, QRS and QT intervals, and mean QRS axis; then you won't miss anything.

- Beware of the *computer-read ECG*. The ECG interpretation created by the computer is often wrong. In general, computer programs are accurate for measuring heart rate and electrical axes, but they do poorly in interpreting intervals, rhythm disturbances, ischemia, and infarction. All ECGs require careful over-reading to avert misdiagnosis and possible catastrophic consequences.

- Don't interpret an ECG without reference to prior tracings. On occasion, a new ECG abnormality can "erase" a previously existing one. A comparison also allows you to date specific abnormalities and may have important therapeutic implications.

- All ECG diagnoses must be made in light of the total clinical picture. The accuracy of ECG interpretation is greatly improved when appropriate clinical information (e.g., patient's age, gender, presenting symptoms, and list of pertinent medications) is provided, and any ECG abnormalities detected can then be correlated with the other clinical data. For example, diffuse concave ST segment elevation in a young asymptomatic patient is likely to represent early repolarization (a normal variant), whereas the same finding in a patient with chest pain and a friction rub is more likely to represent acute pericarditis. Furthermore, lateral ST segment depression can mean different things in the settings of acute chest pain, hypertension, or digoxin therapy. Keep in mind that, along with the clinical history, the ECG is still the simplest, most readily available and inexpensive tool in the early diagnosis of acute ST elevation MI.

* * *

8

Specialized ECG-Based Tools And Techniques

Specialized ECG-based tools and techniques are playing an increasingly prominent role in the evaluation and management of the cardiac patient, particularly those who present with chest pain, palpitations, dizziness, or syncope. Although the standard 12-lead ECG provides important information about the heart, it may not adequately "pick up" all cardiac conditions. Indeed, some individuals with heart disease may have a normal resting ECG. On occasion, a problematic ECG may only register during daily activities, or while the patient is experiencing symptoms. In these instances, ambulatory ECG (Holter) monitoring and event recording, tilt table testing, and/or exercise ECG stress testing may be helpful.

Before any test or procedure is ordered, however, you should decide whether the information provided is sufficiently important to justify its potential risk or expense, and if the results will influence your management decision. In general, the more complicated, invasive, and expensive tests (e.g., electrophysiologic studies [EPS]), should be reserved for patients who have a higher chance of having significant heart disease and for those in whom the results of simpler, noninvasive, and less costly methods do not elicit a clear-cut answer.

When used appropriately, specialized ECG-based techniques supplement the information provided by the standard 12-lead ECG and enhance the diagnostic and therapeutic options available to you when caring for the patient with known or suspected cardiovascular disease.

Figure 8-1 summarizes the clinical indications and practical applications of the most common noninvasive and invasive ECG-based techniques used in medicine and cardiology today.

Ambulatory ECG (Holter) Monitoring

The resting 12-lead ECG records the heart's electrical activity over a short (10 second) period of time. Ambulatory ECG (Holter) monitoring is a useful non-invasive technique to detect arrhythmias and other ECG abnormalities during an extended period of time. Electrodes placed on the body surface record the ECG continuously over a 24 to 48-hour period.

Figure 8-2. Left. An ambulatory ECG (Holter) monitor is a portable device that can store a complete record of the heart's electrical activity over a 24 to 48 hour period of time.

Right. A patient diary allows correlation between symptoms (e.g., palpitations, dizziness, syncope) and heart rate and rhythm. Top strip: SVT; 2nd strip: PVCs; 3rd strip: NSR; bottom strip: VT.

Holter monitoring is also useful in:

- The evaluation of *episodic chest pain* suspicious for exertional (ST segment depression) or rest-related, variant or Prinzmetal's (ST segment elevation) angina

FIGURE 8-1
SPECIALIZED ECG-BASED TOOLS AND TECHNIQUES

Technique	Clinical Indications	Practical Applications
Ambulatory ECG (Holter) monitoring	Documents frequent tachy and/or bradyarrhythmias and conduction disturbances.	Correlation of symptoms (e.g., patients with unexplained palpitations, dizziness, syncope) possibly related to rhythm or conduction disturbance. Helps assess therapeutic response (e.g., antiarrhythmic drugs, pacemaker and ICD function, catheter ablation).
Event recording	Detects episodic paroxysmal arrhythmias.	Correlation of symptoms and rhythm abnormalities that are infrequent or unexpected.
Signal-averaged ECG	Detects late potentials in the terminal portion of the QRS complex.	Identifies patients at increased risk for VT or sudden death after MI.
Tilt table testing	Elicits vasodepressor response (↓BP, ↓HR).	Confirms neurocardiogenic (vasovagal) syncope as mechanism in patients without structural heart disease.
Exercise ECG Stress Test	Detects obstructive CAD, identifies severity and extent of ischemia, assesses the need for or adequacy of revascularization.	Helpful in diagnosing the presence and severity of CAD, risk stratification, functional class assessment and prognosis, especially in patients with intermediate probability chest pain, and in patients after MI and before noncardiac surgery.
Electrophysiologic studies (EPS)	Defines conduction system disease, elicits SVT and VT.	Helps in the diagnosis and treatment of patients with severe, life-threatening or hemodynamically important arrhythmias (e.g. catheter ablation, ICD). Measures response to pharmacologic and/or pacing/device intervention.

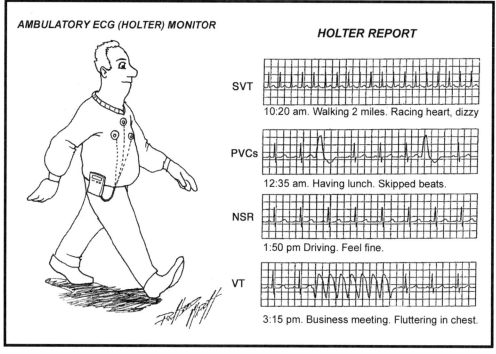

Fig. 8-2.

- The diagnosis of *silent ischemia* (i.e., ischemic ST segment changes on the ECG in the absence of chest pain), although it is of limited specificity
- The assessment of the effectiveness or aggravation (proarrhythmic, i.e., arrhythmia exacerbating effect) caused by anti-arrhythmic drugs, cardiac ablation, and/or device (e.g., pacemaker, defibrillator) therapy.

Event Recording

Ambulatory ECG (Holter) monitoring captures the heart's electrical activity over a 24 to 48 hour period. Since many patients will not have symptoms during the monitoring period, a portable monitoring device called an *event recorder* may be used when symptoms suspicious for an arrhythmia occur infrequently. It is typically worn for several weeks and can be activated by the patient when symptoms arise. For patients with very infrequent symptoms, a surgically implanted (subcutaneous) monitoring device called a *loop recorder* is available, which can record the heart's electrical activity over a period of months to years.

Tilt-Table Testing

Head up tilt-table testing can be a useful noninvasive diagnostic tool in evaluating those patients with suspected vasovagal (neurocardiogenic) syncope. In the latter, vagal tone increases and sympathetic tone decreases on the upright posture, leading to hypotension (secondary to vasodilation) and/or bradycardia along with syncope or presyncope (a feeling that syncope is imminent). This testing is particularly helpful in patients with no evidence of associated heart disease by history, physical examination, ECG, or other noninvasive testing. The pathophysiologic mechanism involves increased venous blood pooling in the lower extremities, decreased venous return, and ventricular filling. This, in turn, causes vigorous myocardial contraction and activation of ventricular mechanoreceptors, which leads to increased vagal tone and decreased sympathetic tone.

Figure 8-3. Left. Tilt-table testing in a patient with neurocardiogenic syncope. The tilt-table test is designed to provoke a syncopal event while the patient's heart rate, rhythm and blood pressure response is closely monitored.

Right. When syncope or presyncope related to hypotension or bradycardia occurs during upright tilt, the test is considered positive, and the patient is returned to the supine position. A baseline shows supine heart rate and blood pressure (**top tracing**). In this case, after 22 min. of upright tilt, BP falls to 70/25 mmHg, heart rate slows, and full syncope occurs (**bottom tracing**) (courtesy of Dr. Albert A. Del Negro).

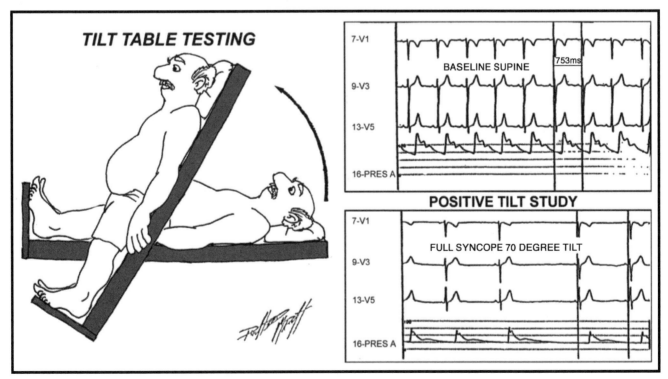

Fig. 8-3.

Exercise ECG Stress Testing

Exercise ECG stress testing is one of the most helpful and widely available noninvasive tools in cardiology. The most common indications for stress testing include establishing a diagnosis of CAD in patients with chest pain, assessing prognosis and functional capacity in patients with stable angina or after an MI, evaluating exercise-induced arrhythmias, and assessing for ischemia after myocardial revascularization (PCI, CABG).

In the standard ECG stress test (Bruce protocol), the patient exercises for 3-minute intervals at increasing speed and incline on a motorized treadmill while being monitored for symptoms during the test, peak heart rate achieved, BP, and ECG response (specifically ST segment displacement, its magnitude, time of onset, and resolution), arrhythmias, and exercise capacity.

Figure 8-4. During or immediately after exercise stress testing, horizontal or downsloping ST depression ≥1 mm 0.08 sec after the J point (the junction of the S wave and ST segment) is predictive of CAD.

Right. Note, in this case, the horizontal and downsloping ST segment depression occurring early and persisting 5 minutes into the recovery period, consistent with a markedly positive response for ischemia, as may be seen in patients with left main or triple vessel CAD.

The diagnostic accuracy of exercise testing in the detection of significant CAD improves from a mean sensitivity of ~65% (lowest in single vessel disease, highest in multivessel disease) to the 85-90% range, by combining exercise testing with nuclear or echo imaging. Keep in mind that "false positive" exercise-induced ST segment changes (i.e., not due to myocardial ischemia) are commonly seen with pre-existing ST segment depression >1 mm at rest, the presence of LV hypertrophy with "strain" pattern, LBBB, paced ventricular rhythm, WPW syndrome, and digitalis therapy. In these instances, adjunctive nuclear (perfusion) or echo (regional wall motion) imaging may be useful in detecting signs of ischemia and localizing the ischemic territory involved.

Signal-Averaged ECG

In certain settings (e.g., following an acute MI) a relatively simple, noninvasive, computerized technique known as the signal-averaged ECG (SAECG) averages multiple QRS complexes, eliminates artifactual "noise," and thus may detect low amplitude electrical signals from the heart called *late potentials* in the terminal portion of the QRS complex. These late potentials are generated by asynchronous conduction through ischemic/fibrotic myocardium. They serve as a helpful clue in identifying

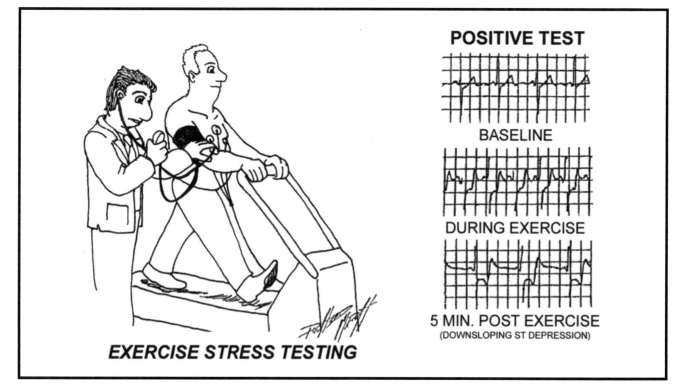

POSITIVE TEST

BASELINE

DURING EXERCISE

5 MIN. POST EXERCISE
(DOWNSLOPING ST DEPRESSION)

EXERCISE STRESS TESTING

Fig. 8-4.

patients at an increased risk for sudden death from sustained ventricular arrhythmias (due to reentrant circuits), especially those with depressed LV function and poor ejection fractions (<40%).

Figure 8-5. Left. Abnormal signal-averaged ECG demonstrating low amplitude electrical signals called *late potentials* at the end of the QRS. These late potentials are generated by asynchronous conduction through ischemic/fibrotic myocardium.

Right. Mechanism of reentrant VT in a patient with a previous MI. In the peri-infarction area (dark circle), a critically timed premature electrical impulse is conducted down one of two pathways in the ventricular Purkinje fibers (1) but is blocked down the other (2). This impulse not only depolarizes the ventricle, but may also conduct retrograde through the previously blocked pathway, thereby initiating a reentrant VT. The SAECG may provide clues to the presence of such reentrant circuits.

Electrophysiologic Studies (EPS)

Cardiac arrhythmias are often difficult to identify since they may occur intermittently. In many patients, a precise diagnosis may be difficult to obtain with noninvasive techniques. For such an individual, intracardiac electrophysiologic studies (EPS)--using multipolar electrode catheters introduced into either the venous or arterial circulation and advanced to various positions in the heart--allow for the detection and recording of the timing and conduction of electrical impulses (like an "internal ECG"). EPS are

also used for the induction of an arrhythmia and the elucidation of its mechanism and characteristics. These tests are expensive, invasive, and generally not useful in patients without heart disease or an abnormal ECG since the yield is then very low (~10%). EPS should be used only when the information cannot be obtained in any noninvasive way and only if it is likely to alter prognosis or therapy.

Figure 8-6. Left. Schematic representation of the electrophysiological anatomy of the right atrium and ventricle.

Right. Common catheter positions for recording electrical events in the **A.** high right atrium, **B.** His bundle, **C.** RV apex, **D.** RV outflow, and **E.** and **F.** coronary sinus.

Electrophysiologic studies (EPS) are used for inducing, identifying, and clarifying the mechanism of cardiac arrhythmias and conduction disturbances. EPS can be a valuable tool in the evaluation of patients with unexplained syncope or in survivors of sudden cardiac death. EPS can help determine the underlying cause, decide on the appropriate treatment, or quantify risk in patients with known or suspected VT or SVT, especially if catheter ablation of an abnormal pathway or an implantable cardioverter-defibrillator (ICD) is being considered. These tests may help to evaluate sinus node function and uncover an AV conduction abnormality (block in the AV node, His bundle, or bundle branches), and to evaluate the need for a pacemaker that cannot be determined by clinical means alone. EPS may also be useful in revealing reentry circuits at the AV node, and in the evaluation of preexcitation (WPW) syndromes

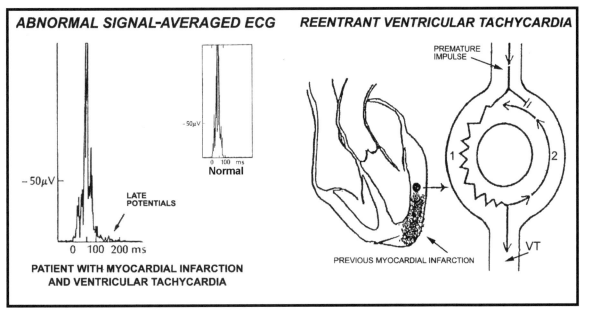

Fig. 8-5.

to map bypass tracts and therapeutically terminate tachyarrhythmias (radiofrequency ablation of an AV nodal or accessory pathway).

Additionally, through programmed electrical stimulation of the ventricle, it can be determined whether VT can be induced in the laboratory under controlled circumstances, and if the implantation of a cardioverter defibrillator is warranted, with or without antiarrhythmic therapy (e.g., amiodarone) or ablation of arrhythmic foci.

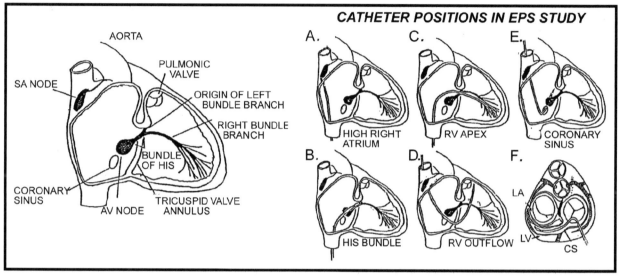

Fig. 8-6.

Appendix A.
Common ECG Findings In Selected Cardiac and Noncardiac Conditions

Below is a table of the common ECG findings in a wide variety of cardiac and noncardiac conditions encountered in everyday clinical practice. Although the most important ECG abnormalities are listed, it remains your responsibility to place each ECG finding in its appropriate context of the clinical situation of an individual patient. The accuracy of ECG interpretation is greatly improved when the total clinical picture is considered, and any prior tracings, if available, are reviewed for comparison.

CLINICAL CONDITION	ECG FINDINGS
Anterior MI	• ST segment elevation and Q waves in the anterior leads (V1-V6). • Sinus tachycardia and atrial and ventricular arrhythmias (associated with LV failure). • Sudden onset distal heart block (Mobitz type II 2nd-degree, complete heart block) and bundle branch block (associated with extensive necrosis).
Inferior MI	• ST segment elevation and Q waves in the inferior leads (II, III, and aVF). • Sinus bradycardia. • Proximal heart block (first-degree, Mobitz type I 2nd-degree [Wenckebach] progressing to complete AV block)–gradual onset, transient AV nodal ischemia.
Posterior MI	• Tall, broad R waves and ST segment depression in leads V1-V3 (mirror image). • ST segment elevation in the posterior leads (V7-V9).
Right Ventricular MI	• Associated with inferior-posterior MI. • ST segment elevation in V1-V2 and right-sided precordial leads (V4R most sensitive). • Bradycardia, AV block.
Heart Failure	• LA enlargement, LV hypertrophy, LBBB, ST-T changes and/or Q waves (myocardial ischemia/infarction pattern), arrhythmias (e.g., atrial fibrillation, VT), low voltage (infiltrative cardiomyopathy e.g., amyloid, pericardial effusion, hypothyroidism).
Dilated Cardiomyopathy	• LA enlargement, non-specific ST-T abnormalities, sinus tachycardia, Q waves, LBBB, low voltage, atrial fibrillation, atrial and ventricular arrhythmias.
Hypertrophic Cardiomyopathy	• LV hypertrophy, deep septal Q waves, anterolateral and inferior "pseudo" infarction pattern, +/- apical giant T wave inversions (apical variant), left axis deviation, LA enlargement, ST-T abnormalities.
Restrictive Cardiomyopathy	• Marked biatrial enlargement, low voltage, pseudo-infarction pattern (Q waves), +/- arrhythmias.
Arrhythmogenic RV Cardiomyopathy	• Incomplete RBBB, epsilon wave (terminal notch in QRS), T wave inversion V1-V3, prolonged QT interval.
Aortic Stenosis	• LV hypertrophy with *strain*. • LBBB also common. • Heart block (rare) from calcific involvement of conduction system.
Aortic Regurgitation	• LV hypertrophy with upright T waves (due to volume overload). • If isolated lesion, NSR common.
Mitral Regurgitation	• LA enlargement. • LV hypertrophy, atrial fibrillation common.
Mitral Stenosis	• LA enlargement (*P mitrale*). • RV hypertrophy and right axis deviation (if pulmonary hypertension is present), atrial fibrillation frequent.
Mitral Valve Prolapse	• ST segment depression and/or T wave abnormalities in inferolateral leads, prolonged QT, PACs, PVCs.
Infective Endocarditis	• May be normal, or show findings of preexisting cardiac disease, e.g., LA/LV or RA/RV hypertrophy or enlargement, new conduction abnormalities (secondary to septal abscess), acute MI (due to coronary artery embolus).
Aortic Dissection	• May be normal. If dissection involves coronary ostia, MI (particularly inferior) may occur.
Acute Pericarditis	• Diffuse concave ST segment elevation (without reciprocal depression) in all leads except aVR and V1, PR segment depression. • Q wave formation does not occur.

Cardiac Tamponade	• Electrical alternans, low voltage (due to large pericardial effusion).
Constrictive Pericarditis	• +/- Low voltage, non-specific ST-T changes, atrial fibrillation.
Hypertension	• LV hypertrophy with *strain*, LA enlargement.
Idiopathic (Primary) Pulmonary Hypertension	• Right axis deviation, RBBB, RA enlargement *(P pulmonale)*, RV hypertrophy.
WPW (Preexcitation) Syndrome	• Short PR interval, delta wave, wide QRS complex.
LGL Syndrome	• Short PR interval, no delta wave, narrow QRS complex.
Brugada Syndrome	• RBBB morphology, ST elevation in precordial leads V1-V2.
Long QT Syndrome	• Prolonged QT interval associated with polymorphic VT *(torsades de pointes)*.
Pulmonary Embolism	• Sinus Tachycardia (most common), S1Q3T3 pattern, RV hypertrophy, right axis deviation, incomplete or complete RBBB.
Chronic Obstructive Pulmonary Disease	• RV hypertrophy, right axis deviation, right atrial enlargement *(P pulmonale)*, low voltage, poor R wave progression (pseudo-anteroseptal infarct), multifocal atrial tachycardia.
LV Aneurysm	• Persistent ST segment elevation in the anterior precordial leads.
Central Nervous System Disease	• Giant T wave inversion *(cerebral T waves)*, long QT interval, sinus bradycardia, prominent U wave.
Hypothermia	• Osborn (J) waves *(camel-hump* sign) proportional to degree of hypothermia, sinus bradycardia, wide QRS complex, prolonged PR and QT interval.
Early Repolarization	• Concave upward ST segment elevation (most often seen in precordial leads), notching of the J point ("fish hook" pattern).
Hypothyroidism (Myxedema)	• Low voltage (associated with pericardial effusion), sinus bradycardia, prolonged PR interval.
Hyperthyroidism	• Sinus tachycardia, atrial fibrillation.
Hyperkalemia	• Tall peaked T waves (may mimic hyperacute MI), flat P waves, wide QRS complexes, "sine wave" pattern (if severe).
Hypokalemia	• Flat T waves, prominent U waves.

Atrial Septal Defect
   Ostium secundum
   Ostium primum
	• RBBB (sometimes incomplete) with right axis deviation.
	 • RBBB (sometimes incomplete) with left axis deviation.

Digitalis Toxicity	• PAT with AV block, bidirectional VT, "regularization" of atrial fibrillation. Concave or "scooped" ST segment depression is due to digitalis effect and is not indicative of digitalis toxicity.
Dextrocardia	• Decreasing R wave amplitude from leads V1-V6. P, QRS, and T waves inverted ("upside down") in leads I and aVL.
Limb Lead Reversal	• P, QRS, and T waves inverted in leads I and aVL, but normal voltage progression in leads V1-V6.

Appendix B.
Practice ECGs: Putting It All Together

ECG interpretation is an important clinical skill to learn and master. Proficiency in the art of ECG interpretation requires commitment and repeated practice. Reading and interpreting as many ECGs as possible, both normal and abnormal, will enable you to gain skill, confidence, and accuracy in diagnosis.

Put your knowledge and skills to the test with the following case-based practice ECGs. In contrast to books with computer-generated ECG tracings, the following practice ECGs are from "real life" ECG recordings. Each practice ECG is preceded by a brief clinical history that places the ECG tracing in its appropriate clinical context. Approach each ECG in an orderly, systematic manner to ensure that important information is not missed. A familiarity with normal ECG values will help you interpret the tracing more rapidly and accurately. (see "Sequence of ECG Interpretation" and "Normal Values" on the inside back cover). After you have read and analyzed the ECGs carefully, compare your findings with the answers provided.

It must be emphasized that ECG interpretation can only be perfected with time and experience. Do not get discouraged; practice is the best teacher!

ECG #1. A 25-year-old male firefighter presents for routine evaluation.

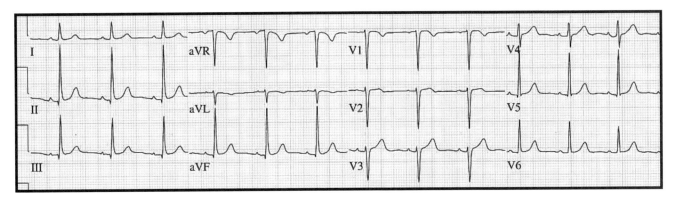

RATE: 75 beats/min. RHYTHM: normal sinus. INTERVALS: PR 0.14, QRS 0.08, QT 0.36 sec. AXIS: + 70°.

INTERPRETATION: Let's analyze the ECG systematically. Note that the calibration mark at the beginning of the tracing is 10 mm tall (i.e., standard calibration). There is a normal heart rate, with a normal P wave preceding each narrow QRS complex, and a normal PR interval, indicating normal sinus rhythm. The QRS width (duration), QRS height (voltage), mean QRS axis, and QT interval are all within normal range. Note that the R wave gradually increases in height in the precordial (chest) leads, in normal fashion. The small q waves seen are normal septal q waves. The ST segment is flat and at the baseline (isoelectric), and the T waves are upright in all leads except in aVR, which is normal. Conclusion – This is a normal 12-lead ECG.

ECG #2. A 67-year-old woman with breast cancer on heart medication presents with "fluttering" in her chest.

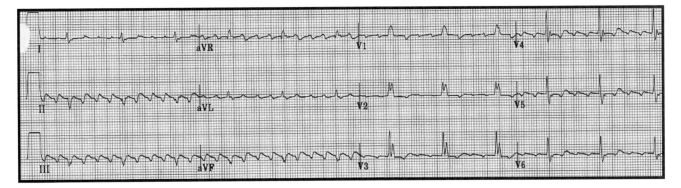

RATE: 70 beats/min. RHYTHM: atrial flutter. INTERVALS: QRS 0.12, QT 0.40 sec. AXIS: - 85°.

INTERPRETATION: This 12-lead ECG demonstrates atrial flutter. Note the typical *sawtooth pattern* of flutter waves along with a fixed AV conduction ratio of 4:1. This patient was treated with a beta blocker. Most untreated atrial flutter has an AV conduction ratio of 2:1, not 4:1. The QRS complexes are low in voltage (due to a malignant pericardial effusion) and are widened with an RSR´ configuration in leads V2-V3 consistent with right bundle branch block (RBBB). Left axis deviation is also present.

ECG #3. A 33-year-old woman with lupus presents with sudden onset of pleuritic-type chest pain.

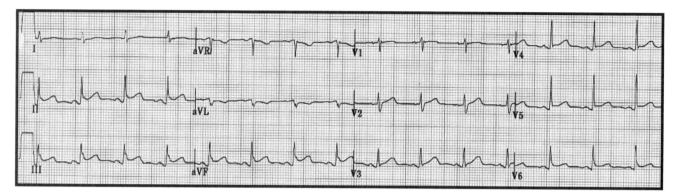

RATE: 90 beats/min. RHYTHM: normal sinus. INTERVALS: PR 0.12, QRS 0.08, QT 0.33 sec. AXIS: + 80°.

INTERPRETATION: Diffuse concave upward (valley-like) ST segment elevation is present and suggests pericarditis. Although early repolarization and an acute injury pattern may also be considered, the presence of concomitant PR segment depression lends further support to the diagnosis of pericarditis. The ST segment elevation should be interpreted in the proper clinical context. This patient presented with acute pleuritic-type chest pain along with a pericardial friction rub and, indeed, had acute pericarditis.

ECG #4. A 62-year-old teacher with a history of myocarditis presents with an "abnormal" ECG.

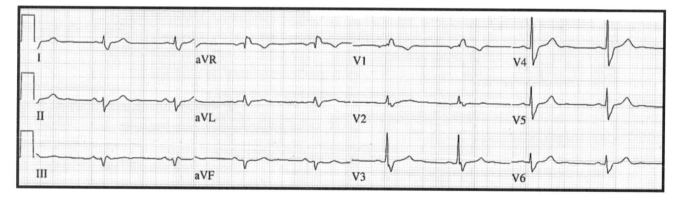

RATE: 52 beats/min. RHYTHM: sinus bradycardia. INTERVALS: PR 0.16, QRS 0.14, QT 0.46 sec. AXIS: - 85°.

INTERPRETATION: The QRS is widened with an rsR´ in lead V1 indicative of RBBB. Left axis deviation is also present. The small q waves in lead I and the small r waves in lead II suggest left anterior hemiblock. The QT interval (corrected for the slow heart rate) is normal (0.43 sec).

ECG #5. An 88-year-old man presents with chronic dyspnea and swollen legs.

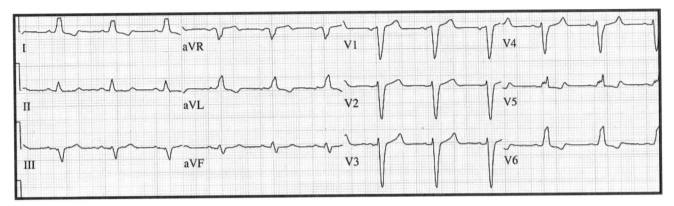

RATE: 70 beats/min. RHYTHM: normal sinus. INTERVALS: PR 0.14, QRS 0.15, QT 0.42 sec. AXIS: - 7°.

INTERPRETATION: The QRS is widened with a notched (RR´) in leads I, V5, and V6 consistent with left bundle branch block (LBBB). The ST segment and T wave abnormalities are secondary to LBBB. LBBB is commonly associated with dilated cardiomyopathy (which is the cause in this case), long-standing hypertension, coronary artery disease, calcific AS, and degenerative conduction system disease.

ECG #6. A 72-year-old man with a prior history of a "heart attack" presents with recurrent chest pain.

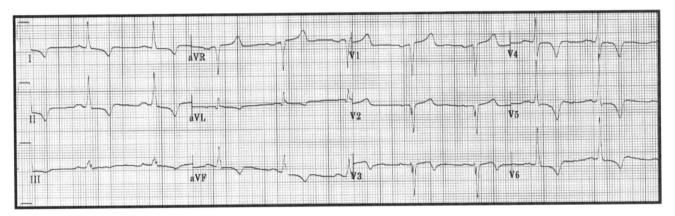

RATE: 59 beats/min. RHYTHM: sinus bradycardia. INTERVALS: PR 0.19, QRS 0.10, QT 0.42 sec. AXIS: + 37°. Left atrial enlargement is indicated by the notched P wave in lead II, and the wide and deep terminal deflection of the P wave in V1.

INTERPRETATION: Pathologic Q waves are present in leads V1-V3 consistent with anteroseptal MI. The ST segment depression and marked T wave inversions are indicative of cardiac ischemia.

ECG #7. A 61-year-old woman presents with a previous history of "heart trouble."

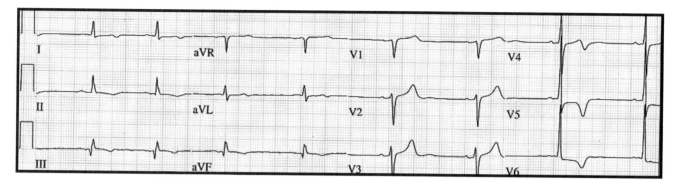

RATE: 47 beats/min. RHYTHM: sinus bradycardia. INTERVALS: PR 0.16, QRS 0.10, QT 0.48 sec. AXIS: + 37°.

INTERPRETATION: The Q waves in leads III and aVF are consistent with an inferior wall MI. ST segment and T wave abnormalities are also present. Because the ST segments and T waves do not demonstrate an acute injury pattern, the MI is old. The QT interval (corrected for the slow heart rate) is normal (0.43 sec).

ECG #8. A 66-year-old man presents with prolonged chest pain.

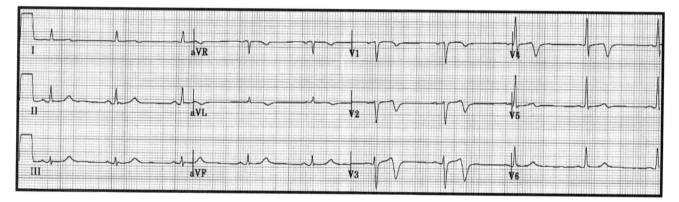

RATE: 56 beats/min. RHYTHM: sinus bradycardia. INTERVALS: PR 0.15, QRS 0.09, QT 0.42 sec. AXIS: + 44°.

INTERPRETATION: T wave inversions are present in the anterolateral leads consistent with ischemia. Patients who present with ischemic chest pain and deep T wave inversions in precordial leads V1-V4 typically have a high-grade stenosis in the proximal left anterior descending coronary artery (so-called *Wellens pattern*).

ECG #9. A 55-year-old man presents for routine evaluation.

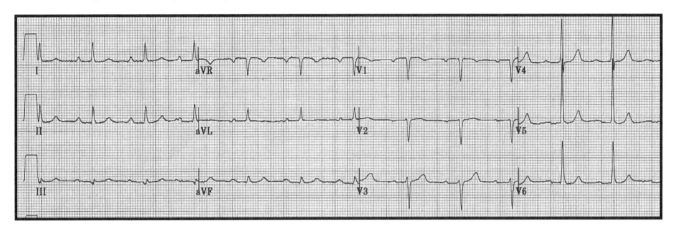

RATE: 73 beats/min. RHYTHM: normal sinus. INTERVALS: PR 0.24, QRS 0.08, QT 0.36 sec. AXIS: + 24°.

INTERPRETATION: The PR interval is prolonged and is indicative of first-degree AV block. Left atrial enlargement is suggested by the notching of the P wave in lead II, and the wide (1mm) and deep (1mm) terminal deflection of the P wave in lead V1.

ECG #10. A 25-year-old football player presents with a history of palpitations and a "racing heart."

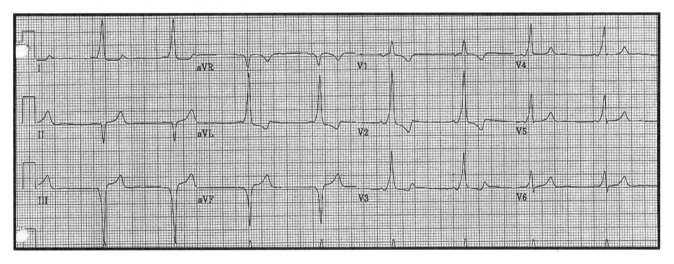

RATE: 53 beats/min. RHYTHM: sinus bradycardia. INTERVALS: PR 0.09, QRS 0.15, QT 0.47 sec. AXIS: - 49° (left axis deviation).

INTERPRETATION: The PR interval is short, the QRS complex is wide, and the initial portion of the QRS is slurred (delta wave) due to the presence of preexcitation (WPW syndrome). There are tall R waves in leads V1-V3 with delta waves in the inferior leads that distort the initial portion of the QRS complex and appear as pseudo-Q waves. WPW syndrome frequently mimics MI and may present a source of erroneous diagnosis unless the delta wave is detected. A left-sided accessory pathway (Type A WPW pattern) causes preexcitation and left to right activation through the heart, which produces the tall R waves in V1, which can mimic posterior MI or right bundle branch block.

ECG #11. A 50-year-old man presents for routine evaluation.

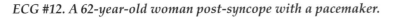

RATE: 50 beats/min. RHYTHM: sinus bradycardia. INTERVALS: PR 0.18, QRS 0.08, QT 0.45 sec. AXIS: - 51°.

INTERPRETATION: Left axis deviation is present. The small q wave in lead I and the small r wave in lead II are consistent with left anterior hemiblock (LAHB). The abnormally small R waves in V2 to V4 (poor R wave progression) are associated with left anterior hemiblock due to the reduction of the initial anterior forces. The QT interval (corrected for the slow heart rate) is normal.

ECG #12. A 62-year-old woman post-syncope with a pacemaker.

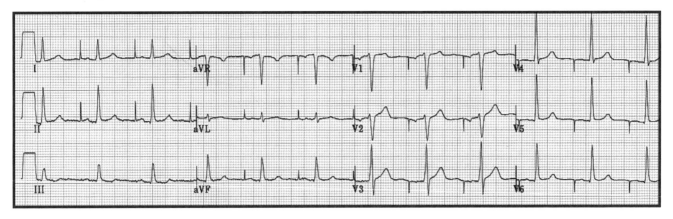

RATE: 69 beats/min. RHYTHM: electronic atrial pacemaker. INTERVALS: PR 0.23, QRS 0.10, QT 0.37 sec. AXIS: + 51°.

INTERPRETATION: There are pacing spikes before each P wave followed by native QRS complexes, consistent with atrial paced rhythm. The PR interval is prolonged and is indicative of first-degree AV block. This patient has a dual chamber (DDD) pacemaker with leads in the right atrium and right ventricle. The pacemaker has dual chamber sensing and pacing capabilities, and can be inhibited from pacing the ventricle if it senses a native QRS, as revealed in this 12- lead ECG.

ECG #13. An 80-year-old man presents with a history of a pacemaker for syncope.

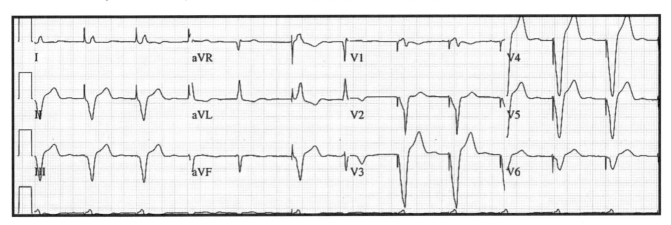

ECG 13A. 12-lead

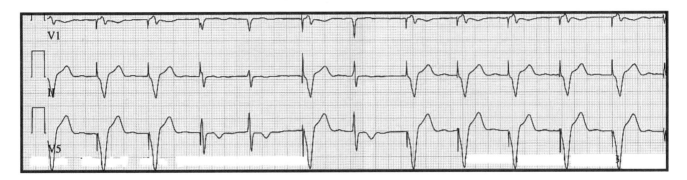

ECG 13B. Rhythm strip

RATE: 72 beats/min. RHYTHM: electronic ventricular pacemaker. INTERVALS: QRS 0.19, QT 0.46 sec. AXIS: -28°.

INTERPRETATION: No P waves are visible in this patient with underlying atrial fibrillation and a demand ventricular (VVI) pacemaker. There are pacing spikes before each wide QRS complex consistent with ventricular paced rhythm. The QRS has a left bundle branch block pattern indicating a right ventricular location of the pacing electrode.

ECG #14. A 72-year-old man presents with several hours of chest pain.

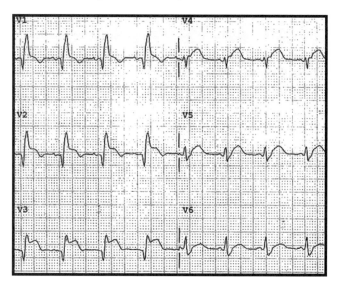

INTERPRETATION: The precordial leads V1-V3 show an acute anterior wall MI with right bundle branch block (an electrical complication of septal infarction). The presence of an acute anterior wall MI is usually easy to recognize because the appearance of Q waves and ST segment elevation in the anterior leads is not altered by the RBBB. Note the first *rabbit ear* is replaced by pathologic Q waves in leads V1-V3. The ST segments are elevated (convex upward) indicative of an acute injury pattern.

ECG #15. A 45-year-old man presents with a history of exertional chest pain, shortness of breath, and syncope due to severe aortic stenosis.

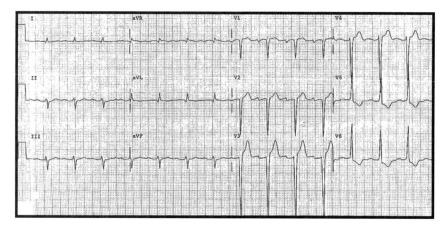

RATE: 90 beats/min. RHYTHM: normal sinus. INTERVALS: PR 0.24 (first degree AV block), QRS 0.11, QT 0.43 sec. AXIS: - 60° (left axis deviation).

INTERPRETATION: This 12-lead ECG demonstrates LV hypertrophy (prominent voltage in chest leads) due to pressure overload of the left ventricle from severe outflow tract obstruction. The ST segment depression and T wave inversion in leads V5 and V6 are secondary to abnormal repolarization (LV *strain pattern*). Poor R wave progression in leads V1 to V4 is also caused by LV hypertrophy. Left atrial enlargement (notched P waves in lead II along with wide and deep terminal deflection of P waves in lead V1) and left axis deviation, common features of LV hypertrophy, are present as well. Although the QS pattern (a single negative wave with no R wave to distinguish whether the deflection is a Q or an S wave) in the right precordial leads raises the possibility of an anteroseptal MI, it is not unusual for LV hypertrophy by itself to present this way.

ECG #16. A 52-year-old male business executive presents with several hours of crushing chest pain.

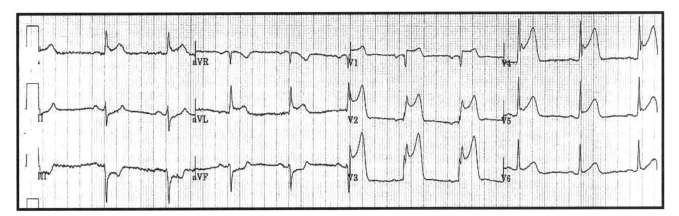

RATE: 62 beats/min. RHYTHM: normal sinus. INTERVALS: PR 0.16, QRS 0.09, QT 0.39 sec. AXIS: - 44° (left axis deviation).

INTERPRETATION: There is marked ST segment elevation in leads I, aVL, V1-V6 (with reciprocal ST segment depression in leads II, III, and aVF) consistent with an acute anterolateral MI. The presence of ST segment elevation in lead V1 is a subtle clue to occlusion of the LAD coronary artery proximal to the first septal perforator branch.

ECG #17. A 70-year-old woman presents with a prior prolonged episode of severe "indigestion" that occurred several months ago.

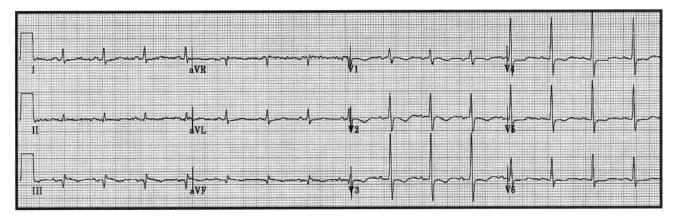

RATE: 92 beats/min. RHYTHM: normal sinus. INTERVALS: PR 0.15, QRS 0.09, QT 0.35 sec. AXIS: + 5°.

INTERPRETATION: Q waves are present in leads II, III, and aVF consistent with an inferior wall MI. The tall R waves in leads V1 and V2 indicate posterior MI involvement as well. These R waves are inverted mirror images of Q waves generated in the posterior wall, which are not seen in the 12-lead ECG. The MI is an old one, because the ST segments do not demonstrate an acute injury pattern.

ECG #18. A 60-year-old man presents with several hours of severe chest pain and diaphoresis.

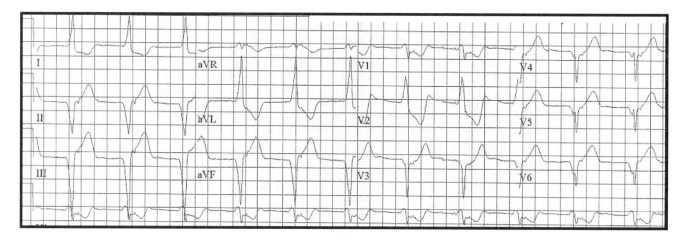

ECG 18A. Early

ECG 18B. Later

Early ECG, 18A: RATE: 63 beats/min. RHYTHM: normal sinus. INTERVALS: PR 0.21 (first-degree AV block), QRS 0.10, QT 0.39 sec. AXIS: + 59°.

INTERPRETATION: Pathologic Q waves are present in leads II, III, aVF, and V4-V6 consistent with an inferolateral MI. The tall R wave in V2 is indicative of posterior wall involvement as well. There is ST segment elevation (acute injury pattern) in the inferolateral leads indicating that this is an acute MI.

Later ECG, 18B: The patient was treated with thrombolytic therapy. Note the appearance of accelerated idioventricular rhythm (AIVR), so-called *slow ventricular tachycardia*, an arrhythmia that often signals reperfusion of the occluded culprit vessel (which in this case, was a large dominant right coronary artery).

ECG #19. A 68-year-old man presents with a history of chest pain one month ago.

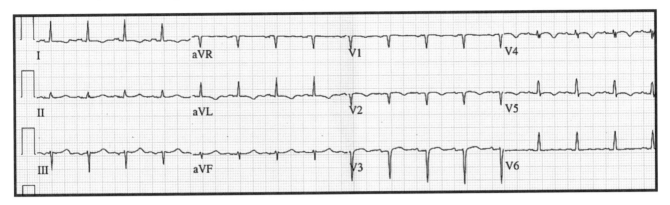

RATE: 99 beats/min. RHYTHM: normal sinus. INTERVALS: PR 0.15, QRS 0.06, QT 0.32 sec. AXIS: - 15°.

INTERPRETATION: Pathologic Q waves are present in leads V1-V3 consistent with an anteroseptal MI. The T wave is inverted in leads I, aVL, V4-V5, and is flat in lead V6, indicative of lateral wall ischemia. The ST segment and T waves do not demonstrate an acute injury pattern, so the MI is old.

ECG #20. A 45-year-old man presents with 3 hours of "crushing" chest pain radiating to his left arm.

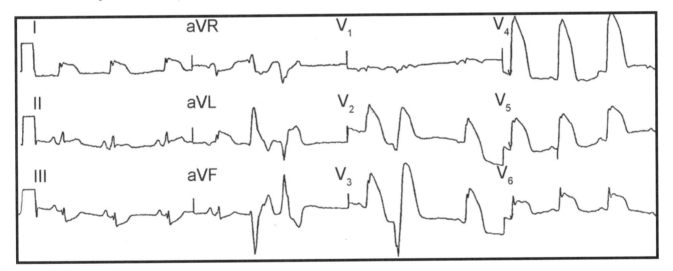

INTERPRETATION: The patient is having an acute anterior MI due to occlusion of the left anterior descending coronary artery. Note the marked *tombstone* ST segment elevation in leads I, aVL, and V1-V6. Multifocal PVCs are also present. This dramatic ST segment elevation is referred to as 'tombstone' because of its appearance and the poor prognosis without rapid intervention.

ECG #21. A 72-year-old man presents with a history of uncontrolled hypertension.

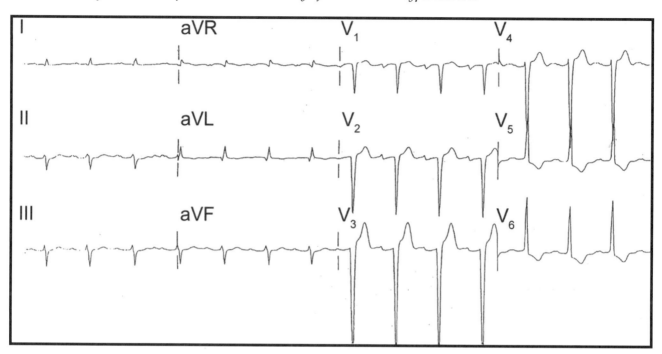

INTERPRETATION: The patient has hypertensive heart disease. Note the increased QRS voltage in the precordial leads with ST segment depression (LV *strain pattern*), left atrial enlargement (biphasic P wave in lead II), and left axis deviation, which are all characteristic features of LV hypertrophy (due to target organ damage). LV hypertrophy with "strain" can be seen with a pressure overloaded LV in a patient with hypertension.

ECG #22. A 60 year-old woman presents with 4 hours of "indigestion," lightheadedness, and sweating.

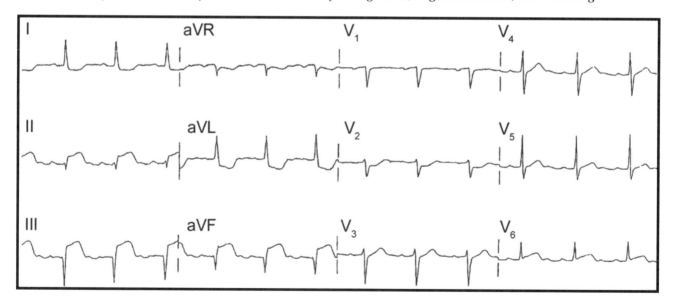

INTERPRETATION: The patient has an acute inferior wall MI due to occlusion of the right coronary artery. Note that the ST segment elevation in the inferior leads (II, III, and aVF) results in reciprocal ST segment depression in leads I and aVL.

ECG #23. A 25-year-old woman complains that her heart has been "racing." The following rhythm disturbance reverted to normal sinus rhythm after carotid sinus massage. What is the diagnosis?

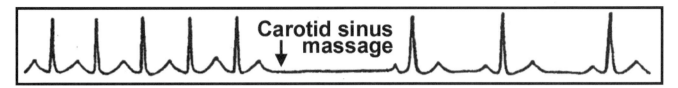

INTERPRETATION: The patient has paroxysmal AV nodal reentrant tachycardia, which is often seen in otherwise healthy young adult females. The reentry circuit is located in the AV node. The atria and ventricles are depolarized simultaneously, and the P waves are hidden in the narrow QRS complexes.

ECG #24. A 28-year-old female presents with a recent syncopal episode after taking an antihistamine, erythromycin, and grapefruit juice for an upper respiratory infection.

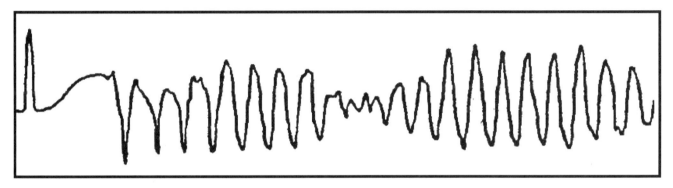

INTERPRETATION: The QT interval is prolonged due to the above combination, and is associated with a dangerously rapid heart rhythm referred to as polymorphic ventricular tachycardia *(torsades de pointes)*. Note alternating negative and positive deflections around the baseline. A premature ventricular complex occurring in the prolonged T wave (so-called *"R on T" phenomenon*) provokes the arrhythmia. *Torsades de pointes* can lead to syncope, ventricular fibrillation, and sudden cardiac death in some cases, if immediate intervention does not occur.

ECG #25. A 62-year-old woman presents with pleuritic chest pain and shortness of breath following recent orthopedic surgery.

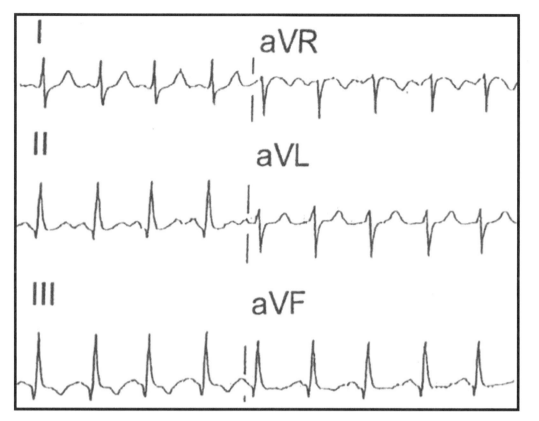

INTERPRETATION: The patient has an acute pulmonary embolism. The ECG findings denote the presence of acute right ventricular overload, which includes right axis deviation and an S1Q3T3 pattern (S wave in lead I, along with a Q wave in lead III and T wave inversion in lead III). Although the S1Q3T3 pattern is a classic sign, it only occurs in about 15% of cases. Sinus tachycardia is the most common ECG finding of a pulmonary embolism.

ECG #26. A 24-year-old ECG technician student practiced taking her first ECG.

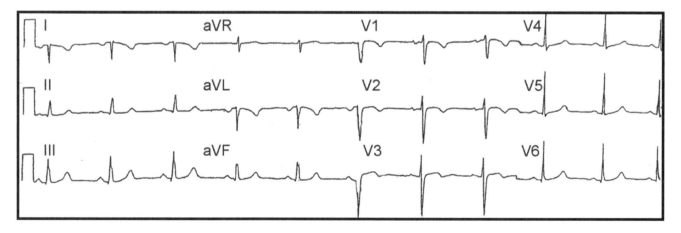

INTERPRETATION: This tracing represents an example of misplaced ECG leads. Note the negative P wave, QRS and T wave in lead I due to right and left arm limb lead reversal. These ECG changes may mimic dextrocardia. However, in contrast to dextrocardia, there is normal R wave progression in the precordial leads.

ECG #27. A 30-year-old woman presents with a history of "fainting spells."

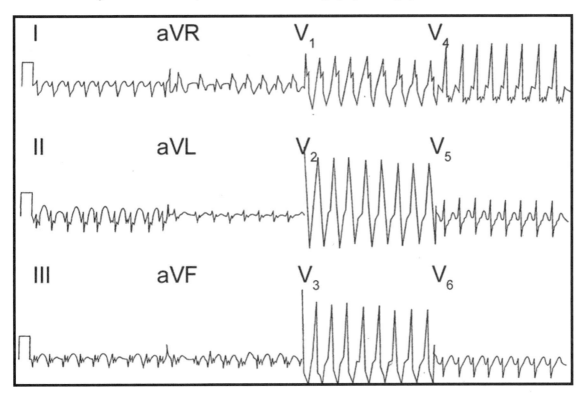

ECG #27A. During a "fainting spell"

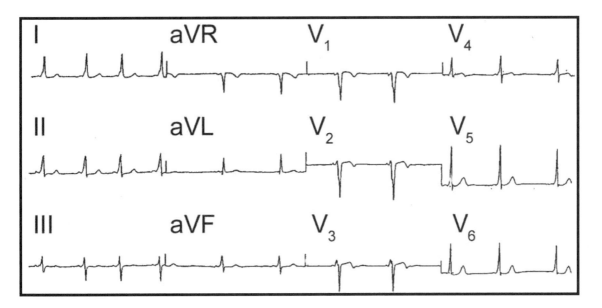

ECG #27B. After a "fainting spell"

INTERPRETATION: The patient has Wolff-Parkinson-White syndrome and rapid (pre-excited) atrial fibrillation, resulting in a bizarre *wackycardia pattern* with a wide QRS complex, very rapid ventricular rate, and irregularly irregular rhythm. After the attack, note the characteristic WPW pattern of short PR interval leading into a delta wave, and wide QRS complex.

ECG #28. A 67-year-old man inadvertently took too much of one of his medications and developed nausea and vomiting, along with blurred "green and yellow" halo vision. Can you name the medication he took?

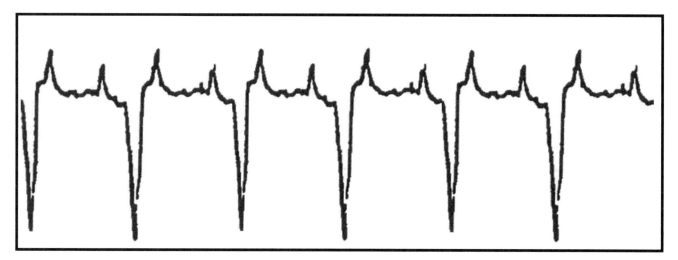

ECG #28A.

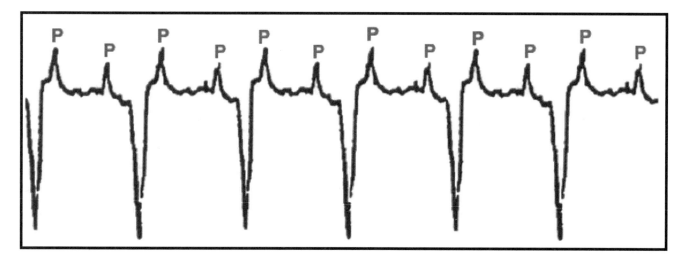

ECG #28B. P waves shown here

INTERPRETATION: The patient overdosed on digitalis. The ECG demonstrates paroxysmal atrial tachycardia with 2:1 block (2 P waves for every QRS complex), which is commonly seen in digitalis toxicity.

ECG #29. A 42-year-old female cigarette smoker with Raynaud's phenomenon presents with chest pain at rest. The following is lead II of her ECG taken before, during, and after the pain.

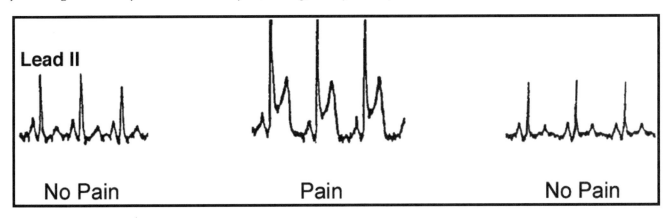

INTERPRETATION: The patient has *variant (Prinzmetal's) angina*. At the onset of chest pain, there is marked ST segment elevation in lead II, due to spasm of the right coronary artery, which returns to baseline as the pain subsides.

ECG #30. A 22-year-old asymptomatic male presents, saying he has been told he had a "heart attack."

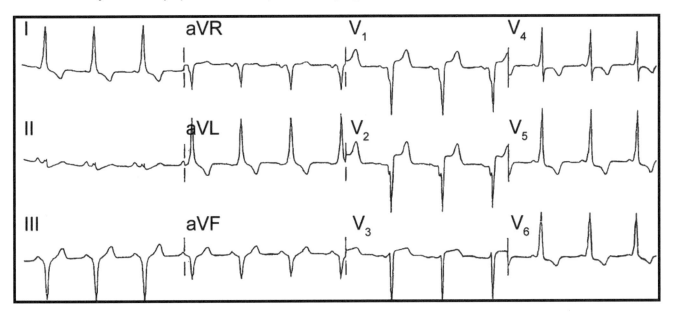

INTERPRETATION: The patient has WPW syndrome, mistakenly diagnosed as an anteroseptal MI due to the presence of delta waves distorting the initial portion of the QRS complexes in the anterior leads. The dominant S wave in leads V1 and V2 indicates a right-sided accessory pathway (Type B WPW pattern). Note the presence of a short PR interval and a wide QRS complex, which are also characteristic of this condition.

ECG #31. The computer "read" this ECG as "undetermined rhythm." Can you determine the rhythm?

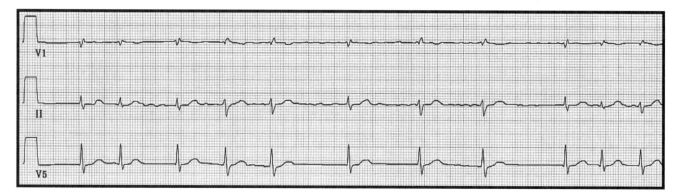

INTERPRETATION: The underlying rhythm is atrial fibrillation. Note the QRS complexes are irregularly irregular, and no organized P waves are seen. Beware of the "computer read" ECG. In general, computer programs do poorly in interpreting rhythm disturbances. All ECGs require careful over-reading to avoid misdiagnosis.

ECG #32. A 65-year-old female presents with weight loss, tremors, and palpitations several months after her thyroid medication was increased.

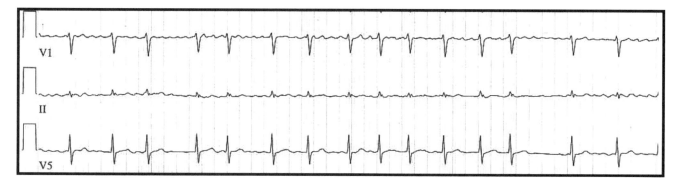

INTERPRETATION: The patient has hyperthyroidism, which is often associated with atrial fibrillation, which in this case is coarse. Note the QRS complexes are irregularly irregular, and no organized P waves are present.

ECG #33. A 62-year-old man presents with severe "heartburn," sweating and dizziness. On physical examination, his BP was 90/60 mmHg, and there was distention of his neck veins and clear lung fields.

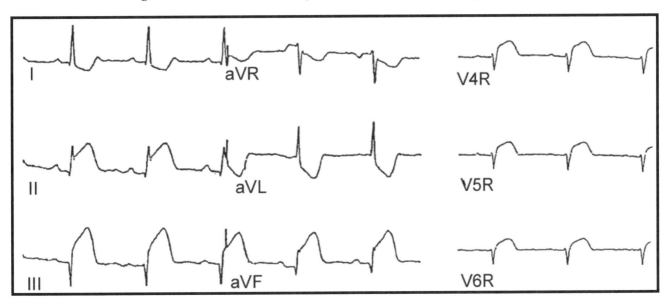

INTERPRETATION: The patient has an acute inferior MI with right ventricular infarction. Note the ST segment elevation in limb leads II, III, and aVF (left), with reciprocal ST segment depression in leads I and aVL, along with ST segment elevation in the right-sided leads V4R-V6R. ST segment elevation in lead III greater than in lead II is a useful clue to occlusion of the proximal right coronary artery.

ECG #34. A 22-year-old African-American female in her third trimester of pregnancy presents with increasing shortness of breath and ankle swelling.

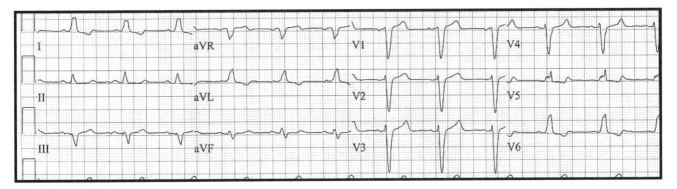

INTERPRETATION: The patient has congestive heart failure caused by a peripartum cardiomyopathy. The 12-lead ECG demonstrates characteristic features of left bundle branch block commonly seen with this condition. Note the wide QRS complex with a broad notched R wave ("M" pattern) in leads I and V5-V6.

ECG #35. An 18-year-old African-American male is trying out for school sports.

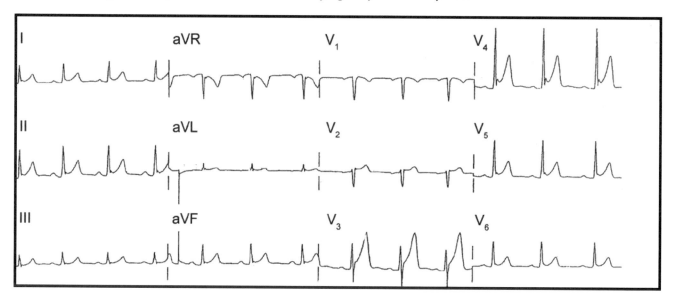

INTERPRETATION: This ECG demonstrates early repolarization, a normal variant frequently present in African-American males and trained athletes. Note the notching in the J point (lead V4) and concave upward (valley-like) ST segment elevation (the so-called *fishhook* appearance).

ECG #36. A 52-year-old male presents to the Emergency Department with palpitations several hours after drinking alcohol.

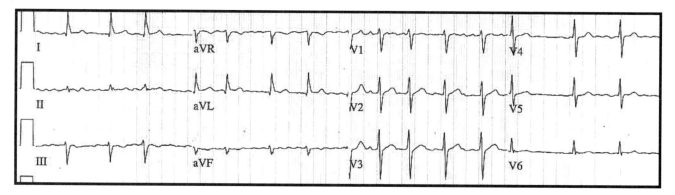

INTERPRETATION: The patient has new onset of atrial fibrillation resulting from the ingestion of alcohol (so-called *holiday heart syndrome).* Note the QRS complexes are irregularly irregular, and no organized P waves are present.

ECG #37. A 55-year-old man is admitted to the hospital after a cardiac arrest from which he was successfully resuscitated. His ECGs over the past several years all looked the same as the following:

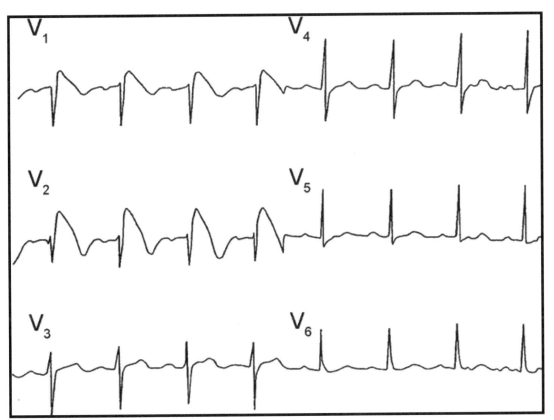

INTERPRETATION: The patient has Brugada syndrome. Note the ST segment elevation in leads V1-V2 along with right bundle branch morphology. The T waves are inverted and the ST segment has a characteristic coved shape. Patients like this may develop ventricular tachycardia, ventricular fibrillation, and sudden cardiac death. The definitive treatment is an implantable cardioverter defibrillator (ICD).

ECG #38. A 66-year-old man presents to the Emergency Department with a recent syncopal episode. The following rhythm strip was recorded on telemetry.

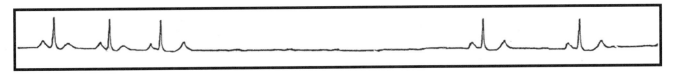

INTERPRETATION: The patient has sick sinus syndrome. Note the prolonged sinus pause. Treatment involves the removal of bradycardia-inducing drugs, if possible, or artificial pacemaker insertion.

ECG #39. A 45-year-old man presents to the Emergency Department with unstable angina. What can you surmise about his coronary anatomy from the following ECG?

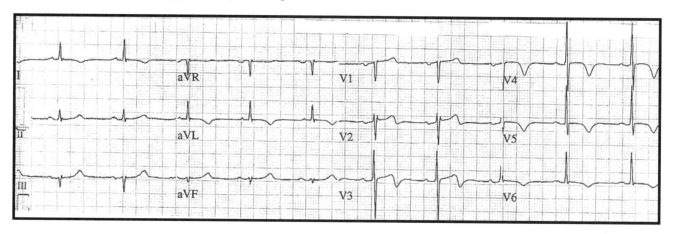

INTERPRETATION: The ECG demonstrates T wave inversions in the anterolateral leads (I, AVL, V2-V6). Coronary arteriography revealed a high-grade lesion in the proximal portion of the left anterior descending coronary artery (so-called *Wellens pattern*). Successful percutaneous coronary intervention was performed.

ECG #40. A 22-year-old female jogger presents for cardiac evaluation. She is asymptomatic.

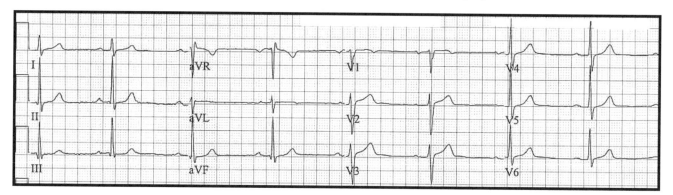

INTERPRETATION: The patient has sinus bradycardia. Resting heart rates in the 50's or even the mid to high 40's are common and is a normal variant in young athletes because of high vagal tone. No treatment is necessary.

ECG #41. An asymptomatic 64-year-old female with a history of palpitations had the following routine resting preoperative ECG.

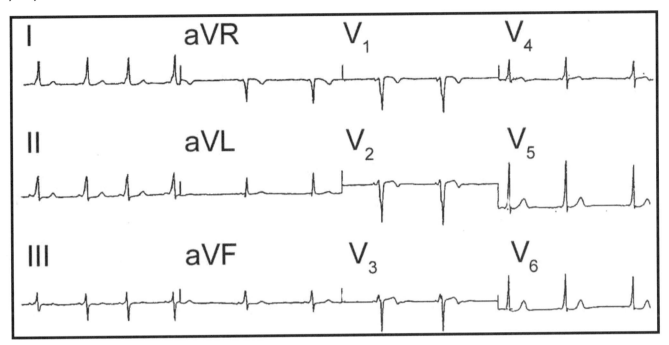

INTERPRETATION: The patient has Wolff-Parkinson-White (WPW) syndrome. Note that the PR interval is short, and the QRS complex has a slurred upstroke (delta wave) because of ventricular preexcitation. Patients with WPW syndrome are at risk for symptomatic AV reentrant tachycardia, a form of paroxysmal SVT involving the accessory pathway. Most patients who are asymptomatic at the time of diagnosis remain asymptomatic.

ECG #42. **A 52-year-old woman presents to the Emergency Department with palpitations and lightheadedness that resolved with carotid sinus massage.**

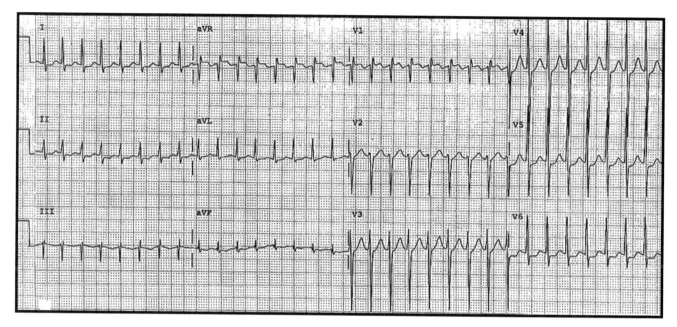

ECG #42A. Symptomatic

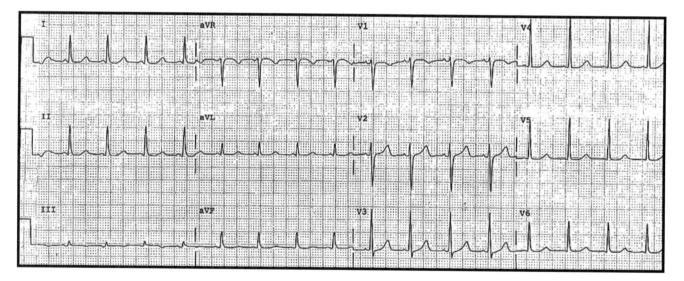

ECG #42B. Asymptomatic

INTERPRETATION: The patient has Lown-Ganong-Levine syndrome. Note the presence of a short PR interval when asymptomatic. Patients with LGL often have symptomatic paroxysmal supraventricular tachycardia (AV nodal reentry tachycardia), seen here with no identifiable P waves (hidden in the QRS complex). AV nodal reentrant tachycardia can be terminated by vagal maneuvers (e.g., carotid sinus massage), adenosine, beta blockers, and rate slowing calcium channel blockers. Catheter ablation is highly effective for symptomatic patients.

ECG #43. A 65-year-old woman involved in a motor vehicle accident presents to the Emergency Department in shock with hypotension, distended neck veins, and distant heart sounds.

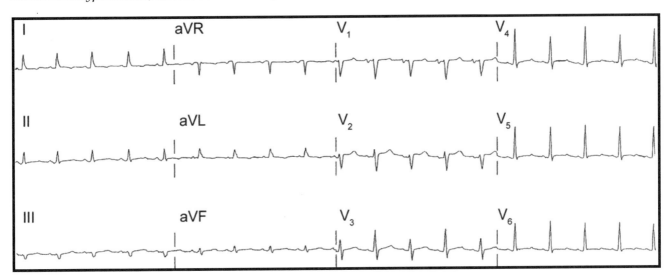

INTERPRETATION: Pericardial tamponade should always be suspected in a patient who presents in shock with hypotension, distended neck veins, and distant heart sounds (so-called *Beck's triad*). The ECG shows low voltage and electrical alternans (alternating ECG complex heights) due to the swinging movement of the heart within a pericardial effusion, and is virtually pathognomonic of cardiac tamponade (which in this case is due to chest trauma). In addition to hemopericardium from chest trauma, other common causes of cardiac tamponade include infectious pericarditis, uremia, and malignant pericardial effusion.

ECG #44. A 25-year-old man with a recent upper respiratory infection presents with pleuritic-type chest pain.

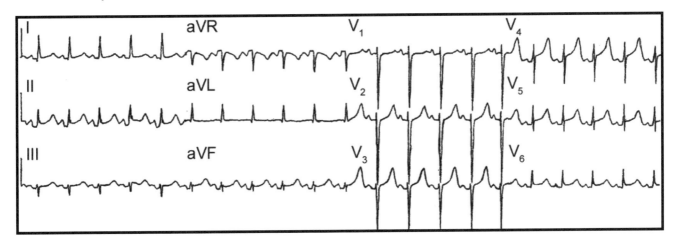

INTERPRETATION: The patient has acute pericarditis. There is diffuse concave upward (valley-like) ST segment elevation in all ECG leads except aVR and V1, along with PR segment depression.

ECG #45. A 65-year-old man with a previous anterior wall MI presents with shortness of breath and palpitations.

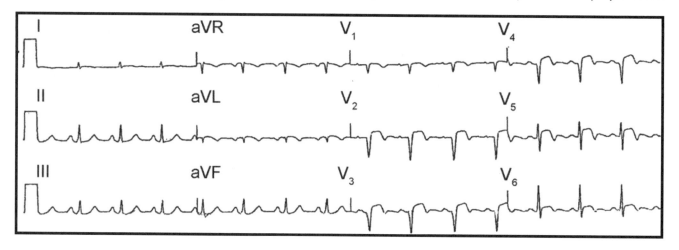

INTERPRETATION: Persistence of both Q waves and ST segment elevation in precordial ECG leads V1-V4 (the chest leads that "look at" the anterior wall of the LV) several weeks or more after an MI provides a clue to the presence of a left ventricular aneurysm resulting from persistent total occlusion of a poorly collateralized LAD coronary artery. LV aneurysms, being non-contractile, can lead to LV dysfunction and symptoms of shortness of breath (heart failure), palpitations (ventricular arrhythmias), and embolic events (due to mural thrombus formation).

ECG #46. A 70-year-old asymptomatic woman presents for routine evaluation.

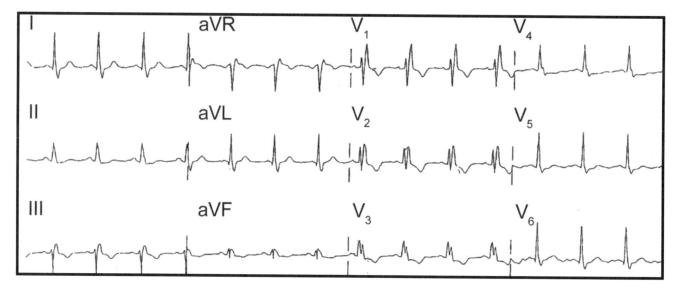

INTERPRETATION: ECG shows right bundle branch block. Note the wide QRS complex with an rSR' or "M" pattern (so-called *rabbit ears*) in leads V1 and V2, along with a wide S wave in leads I, aVL, and V6. Right bundle branch block may occur as a congenital abnormality or present in an acquired fashion. It may be due to conduction system fibrosis, myocardial disease, or myocardial infarction. It is not unusual, however, to detect RBBB in patients with no other clinical evidence of cardiac disease.

ECG #47. A 22-year-old woman with mitral valve prolapse presents with palpitations.

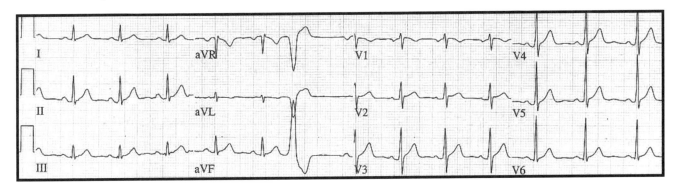

INTERPRETATION: The ECG shows premature ventricular contractions, which commonly occur with this condition. Note that the early beat is wide with a full compensatory pause between narrow beats.

ECG #48. A 72-year-old man presents with a pacemaker.

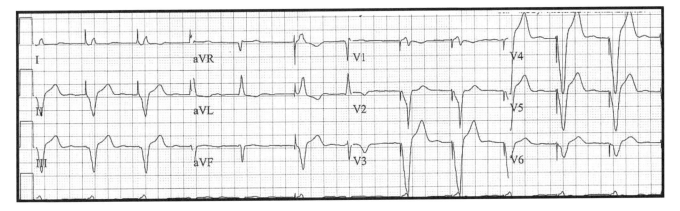

INTERPRETATION: The ECG demonstrates ventricular paced rhythm. Note the left bundle branch block configuration of the paced beats, due to delayed LV stimulation seen with pacing the RV apex, the most common ventricular pacing site.

ECG #49. A 25-year-old female athlete presents for routine evaluation.

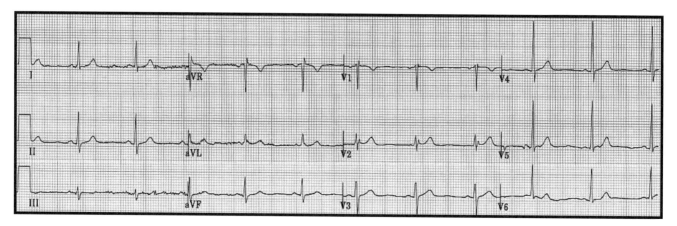

INTERPRETATION: The ECG is normal. Note the rSr' with a narrow QRS complex (incomplete RBBB pattern) in leads V1 and V2, which may be a normal variant.

ECG #50. A 56-year-old business executive presents with recurrent chest pain on exertion.

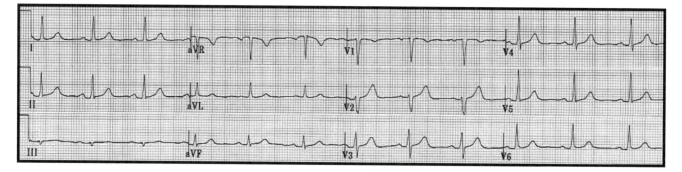

INTERPRETATION: The ECG is normal. This ECG tracing was taken from a patient with stable (exertional) angina pectoris. It is common to find no abnormality in the resting ECG in such patients when no symptoms (and no ischemia) are present.

ECG #51. A 21-year-old asymptomatic female medical student presents with a history of a heart murmur since childhood.

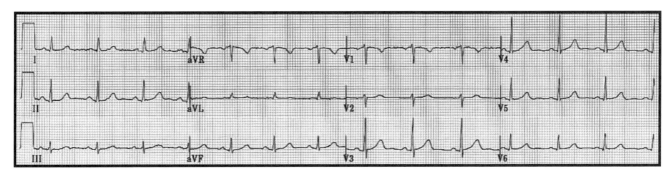

INTERPRETATION: The patient has an innocent systolic murmur. Her ECG is normal

ECG #52. A 21-year-old male athlete with a "heart murmur" since childhood presents with a recent syncopal episode while playing football.

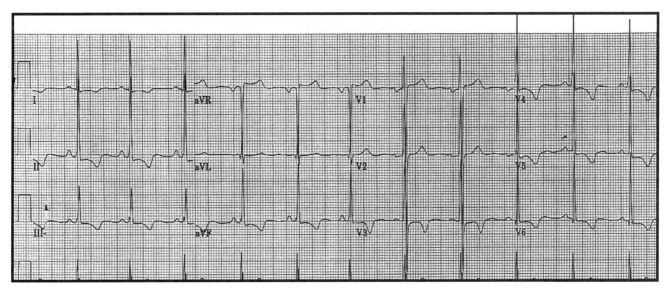

INTERPRETATION: The patient has hypertrophic obstructive cardiomyopathy (HOCM). The ECG shows LV hypertrophy with narrow "septal" Q waves in the lateral leads, left atrial enlargement, and marked ST-T abnormalities.

ECG #53. An 18-year-old male student trying out for high school sports.

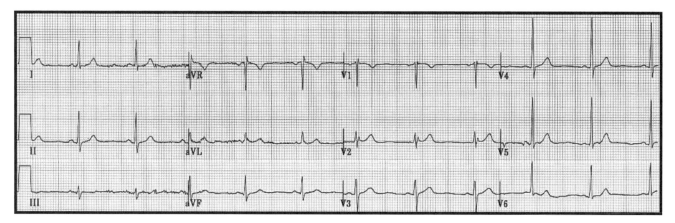

INTERPRETATION: The ECG is normal (which is often the case) in this young healthy athlete.

ECG #54. A 65-year-old man presents with sudden onset of severe "ripping" or "tearing" chest pain radiating to the upper back. He was diagnosed with an acute aortic dissection.

INTERPRETATION: Note that despite this catastrophic event, the ECG is normal. Remember, a very sick patient can have a normal ECG! Always use all of the information available to you and don't rely on the ECG alone. A rare patient with aortic dissection may develop ST segment elevation if the dissection involves the ostium of a coronary artery (particularly the right) with resultant ECG findings of acute inferior MI.

ECG #55. A 59-year-old obese woman presents for cardiac evaluation. She has tried many different diets in her attempt to lose weight and had taken Phen-fen in the past.

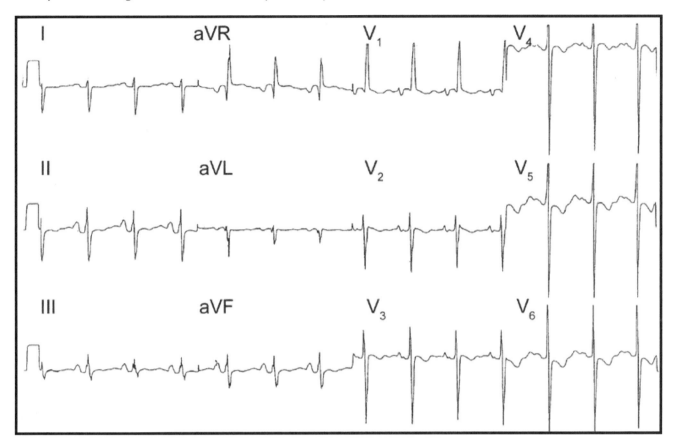

INTERPRETATION: The patient has pulmonary hypertension, which, in this case, is associated with the use of the appetite suppressant drug Phen-fen. The ECG demonstrates RV hypertrophy (tall R wave in lead V1) with persistent S waves and right axis deviation, typically seen in the condition. A tall, peaked P wave ("P pulmonale") is also seen in lead II.

Selected Reading

Aehlert B. *ECGs Made Easy.* 6th ed. St. Louis, MO: Elsevier, 2018

Baltazar RF. *Basic and Bedside Electrocardiography.* Philadelphia, PA: Lippincott Williams & Wilkins, 2009.

Bayes de Luna A. *Basic Electrocardiography: Normal and Abnormal Patterns.* Malden, MA: Wiley-Blackwell, 2007.

Bayes de Luna A. *Clinical Electrocardiography: A Textbook.* Hoboken, NJ: Wiley-Blackwell, 2012.

Chizner MA. *Cardiac Physical Exam Made Ridiculously Simple.* Miami, FL: Medmaster, Inc., 2020.

Chizner, MA, Chizner RE. *Cardiac Drugs Made Ridiculously Simple.* Miami, FL: Medmaster, Inc., 2020.

Chizner MA. *Clinical Cardiology Made Ridiculously Simple.* 5th ed. Miami, FL: MedMaster, Inc., 2020.

Chizner MA (ed). *Classic Teachings in Clinical Cardiology: A Tribute to W. Proctor Harvey, M.D.* Cedar Grove, NJ: Laennec, 1996.

Conover MB. *Understanding Electrocardiography:* 8th Ed. St Louis, MO: Mosby, 2003.

Dubin D. *Rapid Interpretation of EKGs.* 6th ed. Tampa, FL: Cover Publishing, 2000.

Ferry DR. *ECG in 10 Days.* 2nd ed. New York, NY: McGraw Hill Professional Companies, Inc., 2013.

Fuster V, Harrington R, Narula J (eds). *Hurst's The Heart.* 14th ed. New York, NY: McGraw-Hill, 2017.

Garcia T, Holtz N. *Introduction to 12-Lead ECG: The Art of Interpretation.* 2nd ed. Burlington, MA: Jones & Bartlett Learning, 2015.

Goldberger AS, Goldberger ZD, Shrilkin A. *Goldberger's Clinical Electrocardiography: A Simplified Approach.* 8th ed. Philadelphia, PA: Elsevier Saunders, 2013.

Grauer K. *ECG Pocket Brain.* 6th ed. Gainesville, FL: KG/EKG Press, 2014.

Hampton J, Hampton J. *The ECG Made Easy.* 9th ed. Philadelphia, PA: Elsevier, 2019.

Herring, N, Paterson DJ. *Levick's Introduction to Cardiovascular Physiology.* 6th ed. Boca Raton, FL: CRC Press, Taylor & Francis Group, LLC., 2018.

Houghton AR. *Making Sense of the ECG. A Hands-on Guide.* 5th ed. Boca Raton, FL: CRC Press, Taylor & Francis Group, LLC., 2020.

Kenny T. *The Nuts and Bolts of Cardiac Pacing.* 2nd ed. Hoboken, NJ: Wiley Blackwell, 2008.

Kenny T. *The Nuts and Bolts of Paced ECG Interpretation.* Hoboken, NJ: Wiley-Blackwell, 2009.

Klabunde RE. *Cardiovascular Physiology Concepts.* 2nd ed. Baltimore, MD: Lippincott Williams & Wilkins, 2012.

Kusumoto FM. *ECG Interpretation: From Pathophysiology to Clinical Applications.* 2nd ed. New York, NY: Springer Science and Business Media, LLC., 2020

Lilly LS (ed). *Pathophysiology of Heart Disease.* 6th ed. Philadelphia, PA: Lippincott Williams & Wilkins, 2016.

Macfarlane PW, van Oosterom A, Pahlm O, Kligfield P (eds). *Comprehensive Electrocardiology.* 2nd ed. London: Springer Verlag, 2010.

Mattu A, Brady W. *ECGs for the Emergency Physician.* BMJ Books, 2004.

Muniz J. *Sparkson's Illustrated Guide to ECG Interpretation.* 2nd ed. Medcomic, 2019.

Nathanson LA, McClennen S, Safran C, Goldberger AL. *ECG Wave-Maven: Self-Assessment Program for Students and Clinicians.* https://ECG.bidmc.harvard.edu

Nelson WP, Marcus FI. The Electrocardiogram: Diagnostic Clues and Clinical Correlations, in Chizner MA (ed). *Classic Teachings in Clinical Cardiology: A Tribute to W. Proctor Harvey, M.D.* Cedar Grove, NJ: Laennec, 1996.

O'Keefe JH Jr, Hamill SC, Freed MS, et al. *The Complete Guide to ECGs.* 4th ed. Sudbury, MA: Jones & Bartlett Learning, 2017.

Olshansky B, Chung MK, Poguizd SM, et al. *Arrhythmia Essentials.* 2nd ed. Philadelphia, PA: W B Saunders / Elsevier, 2017.

Pappano AJ, Wier WG. *Cardiovascular Physiology.* 11th ed. Philadelphia, PA: Elsevier, 2019.

Roberts DA. *Mastering the 12 Lead ECG.* 2nd ed. New York, NY: Springer Publishing Co., 2021.

Sajjan M. *Learn ECG in a Day: A Systematic Approach.* New Delhi, India: Jaypee Brothers Medical Publishers LTD, 2013.

Scheidt S. *Clinical Symposia. Basic Electrocardiography: Leads, Axes, Arrhythmias* Summit, NJ: Ciba Pharmaceutical Company, 1983.

Scheidt S. *Clinical Symposia. Abnormalities of Electrocardiographic Patterns.* Summit, NJ: Ciba Pharmaceutical Company, 1984

Shade B. *Interpreting ECGs: A Practical Approach.* 3rd ed. New York, NY. McGraw Hill Companies, Inc., 2019.

Smith TW. *Tarascon ECG Pocketbook.* Burlington, MA: Jones & Bartlett Learning, 2013.

Stroobandt RX, Barold SS, Sinnaeve AF. *ECG from Basics to Essentials: Step by Step.* Wiley-Blackwell, 2016.

Surawicz B, Knilans TK. *Chou's Electrocardiography in Clinical Practice.* 6th ed. Philadelphia, PA: Saunders Elsevier, 2008.

Surawicz B, Childers R, Deal BJ, et al. AHA/ACCF/HRS recommendations for the standardization and interpretation of the electrocardiogram (Parts I-VI). J Am Coll Cardiol. 492: 1109-1135, 2007 and 53: 976-1011, 2009.

Thaler MS. *The Only EKG Book You'll Ever Need.* 9th ed. Philadelphia, PA: Wolters Kluwer, 2019.

Wagner GS, Strauss DG. *Marriott's Practical Electrocardiography.* 12th ed. Baltimore, MD: Lippincott Williams & Wilkins, 2014.

Wang K. *Atlas of Electrocardiography.* New Delhi, India: Jaypee Brothers Medical Publishers LTD, 2013.

Wesley K. *Huszar's ECG and 12-Lead Interpretation.* 5th ed. Philadelphia, PA: Elsevier, 2017.

Yanowitz FG. *ECG Learning Center.* http://library.med.Utah.edu\kw\ECG

Zimetbaum PJ, Josephson ME. *Practical Clinical Electrophysiology.* Philadelphia, PA: Lippincott, Williams & Wilkins, 2009.

Zipes D, Jalife J. *Cardiac Electrophysiology: From Cell to Bedside.* 5th ed. Philadelphia, PA: Saunders, 2013.

Zipes DP, Libby P, Bonow RO, Mann DL, Tomaselli GF (eds). *Braunwald's Heart Disease: A Textbook of Cardiovascular Medicine.* 11th ed. Philadelphia, PA: Elsevier, 2019.

Index